Sometimes, illness is a conduit through which we redefine our lives. Such is the case of forty-four-year-old Robert Pensack. Raising Lazarus *is a portrait of life that signals one man's defiance of death, and his physical and emotional resurrection. Through Pensack's existence, we come to consider and value the true wonder of the ordinary in our own lives...*

At age fifteen, Pensack was diagnosed with HCM, an enigmatic heart condition that haunted his family's bloodline for three generations. In order to save himself, he became a doctor—and his own best patient. After undergoing multiple surgeries in his twenties—one which left a hole in his heart—Pensack finally had to have a heart transplant.

While waiting for a donor, Pensack met Dwight Arnan Williams, a writer who—through hundreds of hours of interviews before and after the surgery—collaborated with Pensack to trace this heroic journey to overcome a failing body through the will of the mind. A journey of one brave man confronting the frailty and preciousness of life.

RAISING LAZARUS

ROBERT JON PENSACK, M.D.,
AND DWIGHT ARNAN WILLIAMS

RAISING
LAZARUS

G. P. PUTNAM'S SONS

NEW YORK

The characters in this book are real, but the
names and identifying characteristics of some
have been changed in order to protect their privacy.

Riverhead Books
Published by The Berkley Publishing Group
200 Madison Avenue
New York, New York 10016

The authors gratefully acknowledge permission to reprint the poem
"To Remember Me" by Robert N. Test; reprinted courtesy of The Living Bank.
First published in *The Cincinatti Post*

Putnam edition: September 1994
First Riverhead trade paperback edition: March 1996
Riverhead trade paperback ISBN: 1-57322-500-2
Published simultaneously in Canada.

The Library of Congress has catalogued the Putnam hardcover edition as follows:

Pensack, Robert Jon.
Raising Lazarus / Robert Jon Pensack and Dwight Arnan Williams.
p. cm.
ISBN 0-399-14001-8 (alk. paper)
I. Pensack, Robert Jon—Health. 2. Heart—Hypertrophy—Patients—
United States—Biography. 3. Physicians—United States—Biography.
I. Williams, Dwight Arnan. II. Title.
[DNLM: I. Pensack, Robert Jon. 2. Cardiomyopathy, Hypertrophic—
personal narratives. 3. Heart Transplantation—personal narratives.
4. Physicians—personal narratives. WG280P418r 1994]
RC685.H9P46 1994
362.1'9612'0092—dc20
[B]
DNLM/DLC
for Library of Congress 94-19010 CIP

Printed in the United States of America

10 9 8 7 6 5 4 3 2 1

ACKNOWLEDGMENTS

The writing of this book has been both a catharsis and a re-immersion into many painful memories. I am indebted to more people than I can list here. Many of them appear within these pages.

During my prolonged illness there were many who generously offered loving assistance in the care of my children: Mrs. Julie Gelfond and the staff of BMH Synagogue Preschool; the BMH Synagogue congregation and Rabbi Stanley M. Wagner; Ms. Sam Mask; Ms. Lisa Kurowski; the Berman, Peterson, Dekoven, and Pesch families. Of special note, my eternal thanks to Vicki, Michael, and Chris Carrington.

I must also express my gratitude to the people of Steamboat Springs, Colorado, and to the staff of Routt Memorial Hospital, whose selflessness and kindness were without boundaries. I would also like to single out Larry and Margy Bookman as well as Annie Jeckel for their special help during the time of my family's greatest need.

For spiritual guidance and their genuine concern for my well-being, I want to express my appreciation to Rabbi Mordecai Twerski and Zalman Torneck.

To all of my family members I owe the highest level of gratitude for being there for us: to my father, Harvey, who taught me about tenacity and perseverance, and his wife, Joan Pensack; my sister Laurie Pensack and her husband, Johnnie Dirden; to my brother Richard Pensack for his help and critical editing of the manuscript; to my aunt and uncle, Judy and Irwin Pensack, for a lifetime of support whenever I needed them.

My acknowledgments would not be complete without mentioning my indebtedness to my agents, Mark Joly and Arthur Klebanoff, whose critical advice on literary matters was indispensable.

I would also like to thank my editors at Putnam, Laura Yorke and Eileen Cope, and at Riverhead, Julie Grau and Nicky Weinstock.

My special thanks to Dr. Thomas Starzl for his inspiring and beautifully written foreword as well as his personal interest in my welfare.

Finally, my deepest gratitude goes to my wife, Abbe, whose bravery and undying love for me are documented in these pages.

R.J.P.

I have learned the easy way that the greatest gifts a writer can receive at the beginning of his or her career are a mild sense of confidence and wherewithal; I have been so lucky as to have received both from many people. But it is the love and generosity of my mother, Faith Williams-Heikes, and her husband, J. R. Heikes, that have been most meaningful. Also, my brother Rod and his wife, Kim, along with my sisters Jennifer and Theresa, have made a lot of bad loans through the years based solely on hope, and they need to be thanked.

Without the support and literary judgment of a few friends, this book would have been much less than what it is. I would like to thank the entire staff of the *Steamboat Pilot* newspaper, and in particular John J. Brennan, Joanna Dodder, Toni Bufkin, Suzanne Antinoro, Deb Proper, Keith Kramer, Sean Callahan, and Brad Bolchunos. Other close friends need to be thanked as

ACKNOWLEDGMENTS

well: Steve and Linda Kozler, Amy Williams, Rob House, Trace Reddell, Diane Miesen, Mark and Audry Small, Dick Gottsegen, Richard Pensack, Lisa Skinner, Bruce Daley, Michael Durian, and Thomas Easterling III. I would also like to thank Dr. Thomas Starzl, one of my medical and literary heroes, for writing such a poignant foreword.

I owe one of the greatest debts I've ever incurred to Bob and Abbe Pensack, whose story will never fail to inspire. They will dwell in my heart for the rest of my days.

Finally, I would like to thank our intrepid agent, Mark Joly, and our hardcover editors, Laura Yorke and Eileen Cope. Their literary acumen is equaled only by their kindness and charm. And thank you too, little Harper Bookman.

D.A.W.

Raising Lazarus is dedicated to the thousands of men and women who have thought of others in their hour of deepest grief and given "the gift of life" through organ donation.

This book is further dedicated to my children,
Max Jacob and Miriam Rose,
and my loving wife, Abbe,
without whom Lazarus would never have risen.
R.J.P.

This book is also dedicated to the memory of
Arnan Williams (1932–1991).
D.A.W.

FOREWORD

Raising Lazarus is a book that will be read by a variety of people through different lenses. For those who have not been ill, it will be the grand adventure story of a man who at a young age realized, like Christian in *The Pilgrim's Progress,* that he was condemned to a mortal journey laden with an intolerable burden. The burden would be with him on the athletic playing fields which he loved, follow him to the classrooms, and insinuate itself into the most intimate moments of his private life. He had been sentenced to death by a hereditary taint, without being told the exact moment of the execution. Trapped in a personal dungeon, he searched for a crack in the prison wall that would permit him to escape. For this, he needed accomplices. These come and go through the pages of the book in the form of doctors, nurses, family members, and friends.

The incredible near-death experiences along the way would have crushed or driven mad someone with less resiliency. Instead, Bobby Pensack became Dr. Pensack, drifted to psychiatry, and constructed his harrowing experiences into a framework with which to treat victims of war-related and other kinds of life-threatening stress. He, and they too, suffered from terror, not cowardice. The fear was not of dying, which would have been the easy way out, but of vulnerability. Here is where the healthy reader will leave the one who has been through a Pensack experience. Those who have tasted his vulnerability will remember how they also walked through crowded malls or sat in lecture halls, keeping a physical and emotional distance from others, knowing how easily their fragile shell could be discovered and broken. It is this secret world that Dr. Pensack reveals, in which he fought, first to survive, second to retain his sanity, and above all to be useful.

This book also is an epic of progress in the field of transplantation which dawned in 1962 at almost the same time that Bob Pensack's medical diagnosis was made, and reached full bloom in time to save him thirty years later. Remarkably, he played a role in this evolution by helping to produce one of the antirejection drugs with which he was treated at the time of his greatest need twenty years later. Although none of us knew it when he was working on this project in 1972, the time bomb inside his chest was already ticking. At the end of the countdown, the two transplant surgeons who labored all night to reawaken his sluggish new heart were men who had been taught surgery while I was their chief at the University of Colorado.

The coincidence did not end there. In January 1994, Bob Pensack called me with the news that his transplanted heart had been undergoing recurrent rejections, each episode eating away part of its precious function and requiring dose escalation of his antirejection drugs to levels that were degrading the quality of his new life. He had heard of a new drug, still known by a number (FK-506), developed by us in Pittsburgh but not yet released by the FDA, which was superior to anything previously available. A visit was arranged, and I was startled to see this vital young man for the first time in many years. The drug switch was carried out without incident, followed by a happy phone call a few weeks later reporting that the biopsy was free of rejection. The theme of "physician heal thyself" was intact.

This remarkable book came from the memories of Dr. Robert Pensack, translated through the words of his talented literary collaborator, Mr. Dwight Williams. Those who go through its pages will find the experiences and lessons lingering in their own minds whether or not they have a particular interest in medicine.

THOMAS E. STARZL, M.D., PH.D.

Dr. Starzl is the founder and director of the Pittsburgh Transplantation Institute at the University of Pittsburgh School of Medicine. In 1967 he performed the first successful human liver transplant at the University of Colorado School of Medicine in Denver. He is one of the pioneers in the field of human organ transplantation, and author of The Puzzle People *(1992), his memoirs as a transplant surgeon.*

I sing of warfare, and a man at war.
—VIRGIL,
THE AENEID

I am Lazarus, come from the dead,
Come back to tell you all, I shall tell you all.
—T. S. ELIOT,
"THE LOVE SONG OF J. ALFRED PRUFROCK"

PRELUDE TO A RESURRECTION

I

Hold me in your mind's eye: a forty-two-year-old man lying on his kitchen floor in the aftermath of disease that has haunted a bloodline for three generations. Max, my three-year-old son stands over me, his small arms stiff at his sides, the smooth crown of his forehead crimped in wonder. He casually asks what Daddy's doing on the floor, but I cannot answer him. Apart from the convulsions of my heart and a fist I throw against my chest, I am calm. I feel about me a static serenity, as though time were arrested, my life frozen in the act of collapse. When it comes to facing mortal threat I can say without pride or arrogance that I do it with infinite equanimity; familiarity has bred a measure of acceptance and comfort. So in the dim light of waning con-sciousness I want to take in the face of my son.

Max.

In my field of view he appears large and omnipotent. His feet seem incommensurably wide, his head diminished as though hovering miles above the narrowed shoulders. Time is dilated, somehow congruent with the distorted perspective. I have no fear other than that the parting glimpse of his father will be sadly ironic, a pathetic picture burned into his inchoate memory of Gulliver in the land of Lilliput.

Every now and then the calm is interrupted by the strike of a fist, an involuntary yet learned reflex acquired through a lifetime of provisional survival. It is, seemingly, an act of a third person attempting to coerce the ventricles to synchronize their work. Nausea rushes up like a wave from abdomen to face, sweat pearls along the temples. Eventually Max's face fades, and when it does the spectral memory of my mother assumes its place. It abruptly occurs to me that I have outlived her by eleven years. The same bug in the genetic code that showed itself to her as a young woman has finally crippled me in my manhood. *Blood of my blood, flesh of my blood, memory of my flesh.* It is our family's baneful legacy.

Continuity of thought fades, only to return in brief serried episodes. Visions both real and imagined vanish and are magically replaced by voices and the rumble of nearing feet over the floor. Then, as if out of the ether of unmade history, my wife's face appears above me, startled, with our infant daughter, Miriam, on her hip. She hysterically summons an ambulance on the portable phone, pounding out the numbers with her thumb, the receiver cradled in the valley of her palm. She then sits beside me, asks simple questions, slowly assumes composure, and eventually an erratic rhythm returns to my chest. As she holds a cool dishrag to my forehead I see her eyes are glazed with fear, her voice broken. I try to gather small bits of poise which she instantly picks up on. So long as I lie still and quietly allow this sick heart to stir warm blood through my body, the mind thrives, the senses come alive. Concentration is needed, calm.

For thirty minutes I lie still on my back as if floating on the ocean, warding off intrusions of claustrophobia, breathing with care. Eventually the sound of paramedics' boots rushing up the stairs fills the kitchen. Abbe leads them to where I lie, utterly still but for my blinking eyes. My heart continues to race, but with a coordinated rhythm. A gurney is quickly brought in and set parallel to my body as a circle of faces forms above me. I tell them I'm a doctor, that this is not a typical heart attack, that I know exactly what's going on. Nobody at the hospital knows much about this disease. As if in an attempt to defuse the tension, one of the paramedics asks what my specialty is. As he presses two fingers against my neck, sensing the tentative pulse, I tell him I'm a psychiatrist. "Really?" he says, incredulous, as though thinking, a shrink dying on his kitchen floor before his wife, son and daughter. . . .

They carefully lift me by the shoulders and ankles onto the gurney and haul me down the staircase to the ambulance. Outside it is fall, the valley floor brilliant with color. The autumn sun stands over the distant mountains, the perfect blood orange poised to glide into the jagged purple horizon. I inhale as the stretcher tosses to the rhythm of the paramedics' heavy steps, taking it all in. There is a sad realization that charges this attack with a certain finality. I am on my way to a hospital; I may never be outside again.

I see Abbe's eyes gazing down on me as the sirens come to life. We have a wordless moment together while the hue and cry haunts the distance like a dim memory that has suddenly been awakened in us both. I keep my eyes on her, impressing this picture of my wife in memory, instilling it with meaning. At the hospital friends who are doctors and nurses crowd about the stretcher. I joke with them, make light of it all, though my shaky voice gives me away, then the emergency room doctor asks a suit of questions pertinent to this disease that he knows I live with. The exchange of information is quick, and finally dovetails into questions concerning my sanity. And what can I say about that? "I'm simply trying to keep it all together," I tell him.

A few tests are done in the ER suite, then I'm moved up to a private room at the far end of the hallway. It's a small rural twenty-bed hospital and quiet anyway, but the added seclusion is a display of consideration. Gradually it is decided upon that the arrhythmia was brought on by sleep deprivation, and that I should remain in the hospital for a while because here they have electricity, your best friend during such an attack. Sleep and electricity.

The room quiets once everyone leaves. My wife turns out the light, then lies down in the cool darkness on the bed next to mine. She drifts into sleep while I lie awake watching the steady rise and fall of her sleeping silhouette and listening to the soft whistle of her passing breath. I curl into thought, my mind lost in that state somewhere between sleep and wakefulness. If I close my eyes and allow my mind to trip backward, I can feel the closeness, the nearing of all those malevolent stories, sense my proximity to danger, as though moving into a valley rumored to have been visited by cholera or the plague. The steady ictus of my heart fills my ears. I wonder if this is it, if this has been my trip to the bitter end.

For eight months now I've been waiting on a heart transplant list, reduced every night to gleaning the television channels for the unhappy news of a fatal car wreck, a burglary, a suicide—anything that may yield a clean head wound, leaving the heart unblemished and the brain effectively dead. This seemingly aberrant behavior isn't unique to me. On the contrary it is common among those on heart transplant lists. I know because they have openly shared this with me without pause or shame.

In my case the memory of my mother's blood has manifested itself in my heart, gradually reducing me to an invalid, and finally a cannibal of sorts. The progress of days has led to exile. In order to live I must do so beyond the realm of nature and common human experience, so I have developed a kind of blood-sense. Through it all I have experienced the isolation of those who have seen too much, whose victories were all Pyrrhic victories. What I have come to know with terrifying intimacy isn't something that can be shared around dinner tables. The traumatized Vietnam veteran, the Holocaust survivor with flat, distant eyes—these are my people, those with whom I feel kinship. Mortality, like love, is something that can come to be known only by way of experience. Through a lifetime I have been in the process of dying, consistently surprised when reminded that life is appallingly brief, and briefer still for me. The prospect of an early death has amounted to little more than embarrassment and loneliness, even though the routine of living can be, and usually is, just one goddamn thing after another. A new heart was somehow supposed to be my bloody-red carpet of victory.

2

Imagine yesterday: I see the shadowy indefinite shape of salvation when Abbe takes a phone call from the transplant team at the University Hospital in Denver. In a very calm voice, one of controlled and guarded happiness, Karin Keller, the transplant coordinator, tells us after eight months of waiting that they might have a heart for me. But they aren't certain. Nothing is certain when waiting on a transplant list. She relays that the heart is tentatively assigned to a private Denver hospital, but the surgeon there is currently unavailable. In any event, they want me in a car heading for Denver within fifteen minutes.

At the time we're having neighbors over for dinner. When I hear Abbe say Karin's name, my spine numbs, I know who it is and why she's calling. I spring up from the dinner table, take the phone and ask cryptic questions, most of which she can't yet answer. By way of goodbye, I tell her I'll be in contact by cellular phone during the three-hour drive, and hang up with grave reluctance, a superstitious uneasiness.

To preempt natural inclinations toward panic, I calmly walk to the bathroom to Water Pik my teeth. Peculiar, yes, but that's what I do. As a medical student I learned that the first pulse you take upon entering a medical emergency should be your own. In the absence of grace lies chaos; one needs time to think clearly. But I quickly discover that a jet of water massaging my gums doesn't do it and eventually come undone. Within minutes of coolly setting down the Water Pik, I'm shouting over the cries of our two children when what I need to do is simply get in the car and drive. I have to go and I have to go now. I take them both up in my arms and squeeze hard, muttering an incomprehensible prayer to an incomprehensible god: don't let this be the last time. Then I surrender them to our stunned dinner guests and leave.

With the address book parted in her lap, Abbe makes a series of phone calls to friends and relatives on the cellular phone as we drive. Each time the same response of suppressed glee, offers of assistance and reassurance. But gradually the receiver fills with static as we progress out of range. The inability to remain in contact with the world, the sudden eerie silence, fills the car with a sense of foreboding. Here we are cruising beneath a waxing moon that stands over a vast shadowy forest, the green and orange fluorescent dash lights illuminating our faces in a surreal cast, on our way to a heart transplant.

But the portent is short-lived. In spite of flying in the face of mortality, lying myself down beneath the knife commonly known as heroic medicine with a doctor's awareness of the potential for mishap, I grow optimistic. Fear leaves traceless with the secretion of adrenaline. I'm ecstatic. I want this heart. I convince myself the universe has conspired with me, crisscrossing two ineluctable paths, mine with the dead.

Kremmling, Colorado, the first town on our way, lies sixty miles east of our home in Steamboat Springs. As we descend into the lights, Abbe presses the fluorescent numbers on the phone for the hospital only to find we're still out of range of the cellular network. We stop at a gas station and make the call on a pay phone standing within a shaded rectangle of sodium lights. The call takes a few minutes to transfer through the hospital switchboard and weave a path to Karin. While waiting I watch travelers silently pass in and out of the unnatural light between a bank of fuel pumps and the cashier inside. When I finally reach her she's confident, the urgency in her voice unrestrained.

"The heart's yours," she says. "It's a go."

My heart pounds against the words. I try to speak, but can only manage a rambling thank-you broken by heavy breathing before hanging up.

So we drive. Upon leaving the edge of town the car is at once enveloped in the unanimous night. Abbe asks if I'm scared, and I tell her no, that I feel this is it, tomorrow I will possess a new heart. After twenty-five years with a disease I've felt with the drawing of every breath, I am about to make my grand departure. I will no longer have this disease, having exchanged it for a new set of lesser man-made illnesses. And when I die I will not experience the same death as my mother. I have outlucked the malevolence of god.

The night gradually brightens as we approach the vague glowing dome of Denver city lights. I sense my optimism hedging as we pass along the desolate highway and move in toward the hospital. Perhaps it's that I've forgotten the late hour, as the lonely corridor of highway lights is void of traffic. I feel we don't belong, that we're intruders.

We park near the entrance to the hospital, get my dop kit together and pass through the hydraulic sliding doors. Toward the end of the hall I recognize Dr. Dave Campbell, the head of the heart transplant team, carrying an Igloo picnic cooler as he chats with two other doctors. My thoughts quicken as they turn and crane their necks in recognition of our figures approaching down the hall. They interrupt their conversation and head toward us.

"What's in the cooler there, Dave?" I ask as we come together.

For a moment I wonder if I am looking at a bucket containing my new heart.

"Just my preservatives." He waves the cooler to display its lightness as evidence of his forthcoming nature.

We meet at a narrow section of hallway whereupon Dave sets the cooler down at his feet. He pauses before speaking to emphasize the routine nature of transplant surgery relative to him. Somewhere in the vicinity a man lies brain dead until Dave arrives to harvest his heart, at which point he will be dead in mind and body. But right now Dr. Campbell is talking to me. I am to be put at ease, but can only feign tranquillity. My every impulse is bent on gathering information of every sort on this heart—I want to know everything about it, to master it. I search Dave's face for clues about its quality and the likelihood of it becoming part of my anatomy. That he has paused at all fills me with quiet dread.

"We're on our way to Greeley now," he says. "It was an industrial explosion. A metal door to a heater blew off and hit the fellow in the head. There was massive brain trauma and some to the body. That's what we're concerned about."

"How old's the donor?"

"Thirty. The heart's requiring a little more dopamine than I generally like to see."

The briefing shocks my enthusiasm. A thirty-year-old donor requiring borderline doses of dopamine, a drug that artificially heightens blood pressure for traumatized hearts that don't pump so well.

"They're waiting for you upstairs," he says, his eyes suddenly distant. "I'll call here in an hour and a half to say whether it's a go or not."

We wish one another luck and part. As Abbe and I ascend within the hum of the elevator, my mind rushes over what I've just learned, dismantling the syntax into naked facts: thirty-year-old heart, high levels of dopamine, massive head trauma, industrial accident. Call in an hour and a half.

Abbe asks what I think of this new heart just as the elevator slows and we adjust to the ephemeral loss of gravity.

"No idea. What do you think?"

She tightens her shoulders. "No idea."

They forgo the introductions as we come to the front desk. They know who we are and why we're here. After a battery of requisite questions they send me to a room where a team of nurses and doctors wait in ambush with needles, more questions and a miracle drug derived from a mysterious fungus. They take an EKG, check all twelve cranial nerves, explain what I'll see upon awaking to the cluttered beeping of machines and monitors and tubes protruding from my chest in the ICU. Then they reiterate in stilted legalese that I have given my consent for them to perform this operation, that the only alternative to transplant is to do nothing at all, in which case I will soon die.

The pace of the pre-op procedure is brisk, the tone relaxed yet down-to-business. We're on a stopwatch now. The nurses draw an enormous amount of blood from my needle-shattered forearm while the attending physician comes at me with more questions. When all is completed, a nurse hands me a Dixie cup containing my first dose of cyclosporine, a drug that will keep my body from attacking my new heart, rejecting it, killing it. Taking the drug has symbolic weight as I'll do so for the rest of my life.

"*L'chaim,*" I say in toast to my wife.

After the abbreviated ceremony, the nurse propels me in a wheelchair down the hall to the shower. I scrub with the obsessive care of a surgeon, moving the washcloth from skull to toe. Then comes a knock on the oak bathroom door.

"They're waiting for you down in the OR," a nurse hollers over the noise of pounding water.

Standing in the humid silence, I take a moment and attempt to organize these feelings. The emotional contradictions leave me unarmed, empty of joy or hope. In the murky quiet, the din of my dying heart fills my ears, and I suddenly feel weepy. The tie of progeniture, a disease that binds family. Memory of a withering mother.

Abbe and I head down the long, dim-lit post-op room to wait among dozens of wheelchairs and gurneys. The staff are milling about the OR front desk, all wearing identical greens, sky-blue hair nets and shoe covers. They discuss football, the November elections, music. It's 1:30 A.M., predictably quiet. Though most are familiar faces or acquaintances from medical school, they understand my wife and I want to be alone. I roll alongside her over the polished concrete in the wheelchair, and casually wave as I coast by. Once we're alone I zip around in tight circles in the contraption's familiar lap. I make a tight line around my wife's feet, unconsciously venting excess tension. When anxious I get playful.

Eventually we hear a phone ringing down the hallway. After a moment of stalling I roll out between the metal swinging doors and gaze about for signs of excitement, clues of the last word. A thoracic surgeon I recognize approaches from the front desk, as he sees I think the decision has been made. He gently waves his head. "No word yet from Dave." Another hour passes, an hour later than the anticipated call. Still only silence.

"Are we sure we want this?" Abbe asks.

"What's the alternative?" I say. "Go home and wait?"

I roll away again, forming a figure-eight pattern and a series of tight pirouettes, then glide to the darkened end of the corridor. When I spin around I see a row of dour-faced doctors aligned with Abbe, their eyes fixed on me. I slowly roll toward them, lightly pressing my dampened palms against cold chrome and rubber. The anesthesiologist begins.

"The heart was contused, Bob. Apparently the body suffered considerable trauma in the explosion. Dave didn't like it." The distant hum of a busy hospital comes to the fore.

"We're sorry, Bob," the thoracic surgeon adds. "Believe me, you don't want us transplanting a bad heart into you. Better to wait."

I'm not looking any of them in the eye. I fix on a stethoscope looped about the anesthesiologist's wrist where his large thumbs are hooked over the waistband of his greens. My eyes swim to focus as I lift my head.

They form a line, and each places a soft hand on my shoulder as they pass. Once they leave the room, Abbe takes my head in her hands and says, "It was never your heart."

The hallway just beyond the swinging doors of the OR has taken on the air of a concluded ball game, the teams having shaken hands, the park nearly emptied except for stragglers and clean-up crew. Abbe and I visit for a few minutes, then by way of goodbye I tell them we feel okay about the dry run, perhaps next time, and express regret rather unconvincingly. Once formally discharged, we head for the men's room to dress and are on our way. Odd, it seems, that I'm able to walk out like this—no hassles, no bureaucratic hangups.

We drive through the vacant streets of downtown Denver toward the Hyatt Regency. Suddenly I find there's little to occupy my mind. My eyes follow the liquid patterns of reflected streetlights splayed across the feline curves of parked cars. Warm air pours through the window filling the cab as it rises off concrete and asphalt, releasing a day's collection of sunlight. At the hotel registration desk I take a polished Jonathan apple from a white wicker basket and sink my teeth into its grainy weight. When we come into our room a wall clock reads 3:15 A.M.

Rest doesn't come easily. Abbe sleeps with her arm draped over my waist while my mind rushes through the day's events.

That night the mind lives a secret life of its own, never fully pausing through the small hours in a restorative way. The darkened hotel room is a confusion of half-dreams and opaque reality until the drapes become framed by soft cracks of light. Not long after daybreak I feel Abbe stirring beneath the comforter.

It's nearly noon by the time we're back in the car and winding through the mountains. The day is touched with Indian summer, the foliage steadily ripening then vanishing altogether as the car shunts up the pass toward the Eisenhower Tunnel. I feel a surge of joy mounting as we pass through gray curtains of rain on the vast plains near North Park. None of these emotions takes into consideration that six months ago the chief of cardiology at the hospital told me I had eighteen months to live if they didn't find a heart. It almost happened, I tell myself. Won't be long now. A better heart is on its way. Not until later will I reassess the grim arithmetic.

Max is thrilled when we arrive, his eyes bright with the confidence his parents haven't forsaken him. He speeds about the living room furniture in manic circles, his small legs whirring with the facility of a grasshopper's. Miriam, our sixteen-month-old daughter, absorbs the excitement and claps her small hands as her eyes follow her older brother. A sense of triumph mysteriously underpins our return. Perhaps it's the residuals of relief, perhaps it's the false sense of luck's return to our lives.

Evening comes incrementally. The sun throws a wild spectrum from pink through deep violet across low-hanging cumulus clouds squatting over the western horizon. I wander out onto the deck alone to watch the evolution of colors, to escape the noise of a young household. Standing barefoot on the cool boards I begin to feel the weight of sleepless hours. I step back inside and make a last phone call to a transplant patient in a neighboring town to tell him the latest. He remarks that it's been no holiday in the sun for himself since the transplant. I respond by saying it's all about to happen for me. Then the conversation focuses on the small details of his recovery. As we speak I begin to feel my heart flutter, a tiny storm stirring deep within my chest, something that hasn't happened since the sleepless nights of my residency. The cause, the effect, and my only hope of survival flash through my mind with the urgency that accompanies mortal threat. I allow myself time to absorb the grave circumstances before trying to excuse myself gracefully on the phone. I don't even try to explain, other than by saying I don't feel well, and abruptly hang up. A moment passes as I stand with my hands against the kitchen counter like feeble outriggers, and I go down on one knee and begin beating away at my sternum. Then Max quietly saunters into the kitchen, his concentration focused on my slowly collapsing figure. I am unable to answer to the concern in his soft high voice, and resign myself to affecting the outcome of the elegant battle occurring deep within my heart. Finally I drop down on the other knee, then my back. In my mind's eye I throw up my hands. I want to take in the face of my son. Max.

STREET OF FALLEN WOMEN

3

Our eyes follow the starched white hat as it floats down the corridor dimly lit by a leaning column of colored light falling from a balcony window. The nurse pokes long bony fingers into her tight hair bun, adjusting the pins beneath the hat's sharp creases as she passes us where we sit on lacquered chairs like little gentlemen, our hair thick and shiny with hair trainer.

She ascends the stairs and gently grips the wheelchair handles, then our mother raises a hand and mouths goodbye. The chair cringes as it rolls over the varnished blond oak floor, the frame gently flexing from its curved handles.

The hospital has the quiet air of a museum, with its varnished furniture, waxed floor, the small amplified sounds. Long after they disappear down the narrow hallway we listen to the soft cry of spokes in the giant wheels diminishing through the catacombs. With its severe posture and high back, the wheelchair seems like an apparatus dreamt out of the Holocaust, something designed for an invalid or insect.

But it fits in the somber hospital setting. In April 1955 the sick, I will one day come to understand, either die or go home. Little can be done for the chronically ill. The staff are few, quiet and serene, seldom hurried. A sanatorium, a mausoleum of all hope and desire. One day my brother and I will both come to understand disease as a way of life, mortality as something to be grinned at in the morning while shaving.

We hear the slow metronomic click of our father's wingtips approaching the waiting area where he appears from behind a large potted fern, his eyes dry with mild shock. He gestures for us each to take a hand, and together we wordlessly head toward the sun-brightened door at the end of the corridor. Outside the sun declines into sparse suburban elms, throwing a yellow lateral band over the treetops. We drive under the dark canopy of trees to the rhythmic lap and hum of tires over seams of concrete, every now and then sunbursts come splintering through the blemished windshield.

We pull into our grandparents' long driveway where we're greeted in hushed voices and brows compressed with concern. Immediately we're taken up in our grandfather's arms and whisked up the oak staircase to the guest bedroom where the furniture and fixtures all have the same austere elegance of the Depression era. That we are staying here when we live just down the street holds the faint suggestion of excitement and emergency, as I am only four years old. We get ourselves ready for bed before a tall slender vanity mirror set in a dark oak frame with beveled glass cut into a perfect oval the shape of a woman's face. Four spires extend from the legs of the bed to the ceiling like Asian minarets at each corner of the feather mattress which leaves an impress of the sleeping molded around the figure as perfectly as a snow angel. We sleep side-by-side without touching beneath a heavy handmade quilt while an intermittent breeze lofts the curtains into a shallow arc, cooling the room through the night. We gravitate toward each other in our sleep, unconsciously collecting warmth, and by the first birdlight we're as close as lovers.

Not long after awaking, the ornate and orderly room takes on the bizarre air of calamity that only children can bring. Richard and I begin pummeling each other with pillows, bouncing on the bed and flying about the delicate fixtures. Sleep has induced forgetfulness. We don't hear our father coming up the staircase, as his figure suddenly appears like an apparition filling the doorway. He seems to have lost his balance. He reaches for the doorjamb, slowly and weakly searching for steadiness with limp hands. The utter confusion settles us as he approaches the bed. He sits himself between us, pauses with deep laborious breaths, and says, "Mommy's dead." His jaw juts slightly as if intending to conceal the warm tears sliding down his cheeks within his lower lip. A soft whimpering like that of a wounded animal chortles out from deep within Richard.

At first I am confused, shocked, then feel the sudden burden of sadness. As a four-year-old I'm probably crying because my father and brother are crying. Death is a mere abstraction, it's leaving the house without one's shoes on. But for Richard it is both inevitable and final. I now believe that our respective age difference made a lifelong difference in terms of the impact of our mother's death through our lives. Richard was blindsided at a vulnerable age by what he knew to be irreversible change, while I assumed she would be back once realizing she had forgotten her shoes.

4

Her death has maintained an unnatural clarity, while more recent events are mere distillations of dream and the residue of memory. Childhood has been retained in an abbreviated series of cinematic images, a vessel with the vivid power of impressionism and purest optics: the Gothic woods of summer camp, the sun subdued by the arched foliage of ancient hardwoods, the glazed shine of varnished pineboards that make up the floors of the dining hall, a narrow gametrail zigzagging like a hound's nose through vast forest to the calm surface of a pond reflecting sky. The images are magnified, close in, like a child's face to the moist emerald skin of a captured frog, or a metamorphic rock with a peculiar swirl to its striations discovered on a footpath. The tight perspective is a by-product of the wonder innate to youth.

Yet retrospective adult years have lent incomplete memories a lean and accurate plot. Eight weeks after our mother's death our father takes my brother and me to summer camp in the wooded hills of eastern Pennsylvania where we stay through the summer. I recall the new smell of woodsmoke growing in the air as the car slowly progresses down the drive, the wash gravel lined with dew-soaked moss and bark. Our father parks among dozens of other cars fanned out beneath the oak and hickory, and we unload our bags. I take my father's hand as we follow Richard, trotting off ahead of us down to the noise of the dining hall.

Upon entering through the screen door to the log building I see the children all wear name tags and seem to know one another. So I stand silent at my father's side tugging on his large fingers. Richard cautiously mixes into the noisy crowd, perhaps because he is older, while I stay tight against my father's thigh as he mills about the room and visits with other parents. A widower. The conversation takes place high above me, so I observe the action in morose silence at his side, shunning glances and introductions. An hour or two passes, yet I haven't spoken as I've followed the gentle tug of direction dictated by the hand. As the sun goes down, the room darkens, the lights come on, and parents begin filing out the door after hugging their child who inevitably darts away once released from their arms like a bird from a cage. Dread rises up in me as the crowd thins, and I cling to the trunk of my father's leg.

But his head eventually appears before me, at once sad and stern. Apparently he has been biding his time, hoping I might adapt to the new surroundings. I've been something of a disappointment. He tells me it's time for him to go, that I'll be staying here. My chin retreats into my chest as he says this. A rugged hug, a few muffled words about the value of a strong constitution, and he disappears behind the muted clap of the screen door.

Richard, along with a small group of strangers, lingers at my side while I pause, my blank eyes fixed on the door's wire mesh. Then slowly, forcefully, a scream rises from the small muscles of the abdomen to the dark bore of my mouth, a guttural howl sustained by rage and terror. The crude bawl carries through the humid evening hanging over the sullen camp as my brother tries to comfort me, just as it will resonate forward in latent form through the rest of my life.

•   •   •

There is an indistinct memory of a special guest joining us for dinner in the fall, disparate images that linger in a child's mind. Dad has introduced us once before at an ice-skating rink, but this night is a special occasion. Leaves are laid into the dining room table, the beveled trunks of candlesticks sunk into brass holders, the china brought out. Richard and I dress in slacks, oxfords and matching bow ties. All is done with a spirited haste. The guest arrives at dusk wearing a sweater, along with a glitter of small jewels set in white gold about her face. At her side stands a dark-haired girl wrapped in a woolen knit coat with a red scarf whirled about her neck. I watch them from between the lathed banister spindles at the foot of the staircase as my father fusses over getting their coats off. The woman is stunning in the eyes of my father. Apart from her sheer physical presence, there is a palpable verve in the cadence of her voice, an excitement long absent in our womanless home. Yet my eye is drawn down to eye-level, to the small girl at her side. Her face is compact, something to be appreciated close-up, like a tiny figurine in a curio shop.

That night the dinner table becomes a stage whereupon the woman spins fantastic yarns that appear to leave our father dumbfounded, dizzy with awe. The imagery she sets in motion is larger than life. My ear follows the radical inflections of her voice, my eyes the broad strokes of her arms that accompany the stories. All the while the pale candlelight throws dim flickering shadows across the dining room walls. The imaginary tableau is exotic, her flamboyance and energy overwhelm. Fascination evolves into infatuation.

The woman's name is Florence, her daughter, Laurie. Our father met her on vacation down in Florida at the behest of mutual friends. Their visits to our home gradually will become more frequent through the course of the winter, producing in our household a vague sense of inevitability. At age five I can't articulate precisely what it is that seems inevitable; perhaps it's merely the sense that something covert is afoot. But gradually, imperceptibly and simultaneously our mother's portraits are removed from walls and dressers, her name gently phased out of conversations. There is the residue of memory: late one evening I secretly watch on as my father lifts a photograph of our mother from the mantel. He pauses a moment with solemn reluctance and lays it facedown among a stack of others in a cardboard box. He then brushes away the faint remains of dust on the mantel and stares at the void he has created.

Then one winter evening as we sit down at the dining table with Florence and Laurie, our father delicately lifts his wineglass by the stem and instructs us all to join him in a toast. Until now the atmosphere has been somewhat subdued, as no one has spoken at length or with ease. Only the clatter of cutlery against stoneware interrupted by the awkward speech of our father. As the glasses are raised and hover above the centerpiece our father clears his throat with some difficulty and announces that he and Florence are to be married in March. The delivery is full of ceremony, an attempt at instilling the evening with an air of celebration. Exactly what marriage means is lost on me until it is explained that Florence will now be my mother. Thus, I feel a simple cause for revelry.

In contrast, there are my recollections of Richard as a nervous child through these years. I see him in my imagination attacking his nails with his small white teeth. His fingertips are bloody-red, mutilated already at age seven. Though I don't understand his anxiety, I recognize a peculiar fear coming to bear. Until now I've taken a certain solace in the steady blur of events. The vigorous pace of daily living, as it is regularly interrupted by random happenings, is a lifestyle I languish in. At age five I feel the wild thrill of simple living, a love of the routine. But Richard is already wounded, and it shows prematurely in the soft lines of his face. An eight-year-old is capable of a certain degree of cynicism, a five-year-old generally isn't. Even at this early age I feel Richard has already begun to retreat into an inner sanctum unknown to the rest of the family. While our father entertains in the dining room amid competing voices, hard laughter and rich desserts, Richard often vanishes from the table's perimeter unnoticed. Inevitably I'll find him in his room reading, tending to an intellect that I'll come to fear and admire. It is a kind of legerdemain beyond my comprehension that others in the family will simply come to fear. The fine instrument he will apply to his studies he'll also learn to wield against those he thinks have compromised his feelings. But that will come later.

I recall getting dressed for the wedding that morning in March of 1956. We wear miniature suit coats, elaborately designed yarmulkes and high-polish shoes. I recall my father straightening my tie, the humid odor of his breath against my face as he explains to both of us what this ceremony is all about, and describes lovely scenarios of life afterward. Florence will be our new mother, Laurie our new sister. Our family will be whole again.

5

We are a part of the initial wave of wealthy to flee the cities and gentrify what were once dairy farms and hardwood groves—the original white flight. Newark, with all its gutted warehouses, unsightly industry and comparatively mild crime of 1957, is now a place to be visited or driven through with the windows rolled up. Not long after the wedding the family moves to Livingston, New Jersey, one of America's first suburbs.

For a few years now my father has run a small company that produces hermetically sealed capacitors for the space industry that isn't so small anymore. What began in a factory loft with three employees, a single telephone line and handwritten orders has evolved into a large factory in the posh suburb of Murray Hill. It is now an industry unto itself with small fortunes in the offing for my father and his partner. Thus, with an eye along the skyline and a lazy hand upon the wheel of a sprawling new Packard, our father moves his revised family far from the blight. Today we legitimately lay claim to a unique place in the history of Americana as pilgrims of the modern suburb.

By comparison to our Irvington home, the new house is downright stately. It is also utterly lacking in character: a new American home looking out anonymously on to an unnaturally quiet street and new section of sidewalk from behind a clean topiary line. Rising up before it are nude saplings stabilized by guy-wires staked into a manicured lawn. Other homes are variations on the same theme, though as of yet many lack lawns. Little boxes made of ticky-tacky. On the edge of the development stand tan skeletal structures that evolve overnight into completed homes, their yellow clay yards soon to be smothered by rolls of sod trucked in from the country.

I recall standing with my father one night upon the fresh gray paint of the new porch, his gaze scanning the dying light spreading over the horizon. The distance in his eyes displays a certain pride at having provided so abundantly for his family; he has done well, and as a young man. In the aftermath of the death of a young wife he has not only survived but thrived, something he doubtless attributes to focusing on the present, dealing with the task at hand. No one in Livingston is told of her death. Not long after the move our father legally adopts Laurie from her biological father, and Florence does the same with Richard and me. The preening is complete. The family is whole and tidy, not missing any visible appendages. It is also growing wealthy very quickly.

One summer night, and many more following, our parents meander into the living room after dinner and sit down on the oak piano bench. They call us to join them at the grand piano before we've fully dispersed from the dinner table. As we wander in one by one, their voices mingle with a soft rippling melody. Then Mom strikes a dramatic chord, her fingers fanned out over the keyboard, and out flutters a crooning note from her long delicate neck. The voice is soft at first, then grows fuller and louder. We children are prodded to join in the chorus by Dad as he looks our way and nods abruptly on the note of entry. Eventually the entire family is synchronized to the tune, producing a look of visceral satisfaction in Dad's eyes. We are the Von Trapp Family Singers. At the end of the performance, Dad tells Mom she has a world-class voice. *World class,* he says with the ardent seriousness of a Vegas talent agent.

6

I have another recollection in mind, though it's doubtful ever to have occurred, being too aptly symbolic, too tidy. What most likely was a natural evolution lies magically transformed in the fabric of memory as a singular event. Compression has tempered it with startling poignancy.

At some point, either before or after their wedding, Dad gathers Richard, Laurie and myself around him in the living room. Without speaking he expresses uneasy urgency. He has something to say, nevertheless. In what has been retained with a neo-biblical tone, he tells us that henceforth Florence is Mother and Harvey Father, and henceforth they are to be addressed as such. The anonymous voice represents in my memory some token mandate handed down by god for us to form a family. A Hebrew Brady Bunch. It will take me several years to recognize this imaginary mandate for what it is. The male side of the household never speaks of our mother's death, even privately. It is our sad secret, a tacitly forbidden subject that jeopardizes family stability. Visits with our maternal grandparents become infrequent, and our mutual anguish fades into scattered memory. Whenever we do see them, they smother us with affection. They have lost their daughter, and we are her living memory. Her ghost lives in our blood.

Of course Florence isn't so much our mother as she is our father's wife. She's an elegant wife for a successful young man in his early thirties. She is a woman other men covet: thin, attractive, social, appropriately flirtatious with my father's friends.

Within a few weeks after the wedding it is decided upon that what our family needs is a live-in maid, someone to do the housework. Mom looks into it. She finally chooses Georgia, a black woman from Tupelo, Mississippi, a young single mother who will run a household for cheap, and with a graciousness that appeals to Mom's rather imperious tastes.

I have salvaged an image of Georgia: her face lowers before my eyes, the plump black cheeks and broad hair spanning the periphery of vision, and she smiles, displaying a mouth of great white teeth. She then takes my small hand in hers, gently pumps it and says my name in a shy but resonate southern accent. I lower my eyes but she delicately dips her brow beneath my line of vision. I feel a sudden timidity coming on. My first look into the brown eyes of a black woman.

When she cooks for the family, her manner is especially quaint and stereotypically southern in nature. Oftentimes she will bring out a vast platter of fried chicken followed by a large stoneware bowl of mashed potatoes. There seems to be an observance of small formalities on her part as she glides about the table. Mom and Dad are Mr. and Mrs. Pensack, careful attention has been paid to the sharp creases in the paper napkins. Toward the end of the meal she is mildly praised for her efforts, and in return she is appropriately self-effacing. Coos of praise elicit a "Why, you're too kind, Mr. Pensack," in Georgia's easy voice.

After dinner I often follow the baritone noise of large stainless steel pots bobbing in the kitchen sink. I quietly step up to the open door to observe Georgia from behind, her thick black arms plunging into a steaming mound of broken suds. A soothing hum accompanies her work, a gentle rhythm stirs her body. Such smooth black skin. As she finishes up, she polishes the long neck of the sink spout, washes the counter down with a floppy soap rag, then mops the floor. I watch on until her work is complete. Finally she scans the kitchen once again, and I nonchalantly walk away, listening to her solitary footsteps as they descend into the basement to her improvised room.

Years later I will tell friends my mother is plump and black and lives in the basement. She hums Negro spirituals while baking a Mississippi interpretation of brisket and pets my forehead until I'm asleep. White boy fantasies, they will say. We all have them. And so the calendar of days becomes a mixture of memory and desire, recurring in happy little episodes, days abruptly severed at the ends by intense fevered sleep. Childhood arrives late and departs prematurely, a process I can only describe as an assault on the senses. Early memory is my pome, the precious thing I have collected and preserved, precariously guarded like a child with a robin's egg. Through the years I recall the precise shade of firebrick, the acute angles of the suburban school, the numbing sameness. Four decades later I can still mentally walk the stretch of new sidewalk home to find the house empty but for Georgia and her friend, Mary, another black maid who lives just down the street. They sit in the kitchen, Georgia with her short black arms whitened to the elbow with flour, Mary humming a harmony of bop, a steel mixing bowl sunk into the dress between her knees. From the beginning I am drawn deep into their private society, sensing the happy transfer, the encroaching ache of filial love. The moment my books hit the floor I run a familiar path to the kitchen where my head hits the soft cushion of Georgia's vast bosom.

But in the winter of 1962, when I am twelve years old, Georgia tells my parents she needs to return to Mississippi to raise her daughter. All this time she has been raised by Georgia's mother, and now it is time for her to go. Within a week of the news she packs her bags, a friend picks her up in a battered but dignified Chevrolet, and the car vanishes from between the precise ribbons of sidewalk that line the quiet suburban street. She will not be replaced by anyone constant or permanent.

7

One evening in the summer of 1959 at camp heavy rain clouds mount the pastoral green horizon of oak foliage, and drive a basketball game into the gymnasium. Richard plays hard, his face is flushed with color. The rain clouds usher in a heavy humidity that clings to skin, warming the body. Then midway through the game of half-court, Richard feels a pause deep within his chest. He can't breathe, it is as though an object were lodged at the top of his throat, as though he were drowning in the open air. He begins wheezing like an asthmatic, though he has no known allergies. He stumbles toward the door and steps into the faintly cooler breeze and sprawls himself across the bluegrass, inhaling the rich odor of chlorophyll and humus. He is twelve years old and certain he is about to die. For several long minutes the sensation stays with him, hanging high up in the chest against the throat. Then gradually, very gradually at first, breath mysteriously returns in whispers. He keeps his nose buried in the sod, imagining its odor as a sort of healing balsam to his lungs. A few counselors hover over him, repeating questions as he lies there utterly still but for the awkward cadence of his breathing. After several minutes he rolls over onto his back, looking into an empty patch of sky between rain clouds, and mutters, "I'm all right," though he is scared charmless. He slowly works his way to his feet, is asked if he's sure he's okay, and the episode goes effectively unrecorded. Weeks later, when we finally see our dad, the episode is ancient, forgotten.

Perhaps it is the informal order of the court, the precise black line submerged in lacquer around the perimeter that brilliantly contrasts the disorder at home, or the rhythm of a ball dribbling against concrete and the noise that surrounds the ragged public courts in Newark. Certainly the abrupt sound of tearing silk when the dark leather rushes through a net is part of it. Above all we both know that ultimately it is the identification with black culture.

It is also my brother's sport—a game he plays with a grace beyond his years in middle school and junior high. Then in high school it becomes a forbidden game for obscure reasons. He continues to play illicitly, which colors the game in my imagination, the imagination of a younger brother, with the shade of dissent and insurrection. As my sensibilities mature through time, this poetic fascination with the game remains unaltered.

Every semester a doctor comes to the school for two days to give each student a physical checkup. In the fall of his freshman year Richard stands in line before a door behind which a doctor sits on a round chair like a piano stool in the nurse's station. The checkup is brief, routine and compulsory. There are no dark expectations. When Richard enters the small office and closes the door behind him, he does precisely what the doctor asks. The doctor has conducted thousands of physicals before, perhaps a hundred this morning alone. He checks for hernias, lesions, the ears, nose and throat—basic problems. Then he checks the heart and lungs with a stethoscope. As he holds the cool chrome to Richard's naked back, he asks him to breathe deeply, and Richard does so. He asks him to do this again and again as he floats the stethoscope in a shallow circle over his heart. Time passes.

Richard senses the swift pace of the routine has been broken by the sound of his heart. In the intimate silence of the small room he can hear students chattering on the other side of the door. After several minutes of this the doctor sits up straight, tells Richard he can put his shirt back on, and that he's got a bit of a heart murmur. Nothing to worry about, but he should have his folks take him to the family physician to have it checked. Richard isn't worried, not even very curious. He jams the doctor's note that has been scrawled on personal stationery deep into the hip pocket of his jeans and gives it to Mom and Dad that night at the dinner table. An appointment is made with Dr. Gillette, our family physician, for the following week.

Like the school doctor, Gillette listens to the rhythmic thrusts of moving blood, and, just as the school doctor said, a murmur can be detected, a wheezing stammer against the echo of his laboring heart.

Gillette asks a series of questions: Does he ever feel especially tired on the basketball court? No, not especially. Have you ever felt faint during a hard workout? No, not really. Is there any history of heart disease in the family? Then Dad interjects to answer. "His mother died in fifty-five of an unknown heart ailment."

Ahh.

Then Richard recalls the episode at sleepaway camp, the feeling of breathlessness, that he felt he nearly died. Dad is shocked by Richard's short narrative. Why hadn't he been told? "Forgot," Richard says unapologetically, shrugging his shoulders.

The connection of vague, seemingly disparate events is brought together by Gillette, like a murder mystery. For a moment a chill settles over the room as the plot reveals itself—a ghost in the genes. Then the doctor hands Richard a temporary injunction against playing basketball until the problem is solved, and Dad promises to enforce it. Then Gillette suggests the matter should be looked into further by a cardiac specialist, and my father and brother leave, Richard with the sense that this is much ado about nothing, my father with the conviction that this thing can be nipped in the bud if they act now.

At home Mom is briefed on the visit. She is surprised at the possible source of the problem, but is more or less calm that night. This is something entirely unexpected—the possibility of genetic heart disease. She thinks for a moment, then announces an idea. She has an uncle who is a doctor; he would know who the best in the field are. A single phone call later and Flower Fifth Avenue Hospital in New York City is decided upon.

An uneventful series of weeks passes with Richard immersing himself in books and schoolwork, ostensibly without the game of basketball filling his free time. In PE class he sits alone in the gymnasium, dressed in street clothes with books cupped in his hand while the class plays half-court. But after school he plays subversively on public courts without a net hanging from the rust-colored rim. It is another world in another part of town, a place no one would think to look for him. From time to time I come along to watch and play the forbidden game. His audacity thrills me.

Then one Monday Mom, Dad and Richard leave for Flower Fifth Avenue Hospital in New York City. Their departure is unceremonious enough; Dad tells me they'll be back in two days with the answers to the riddle.

Fifth Avenue in New York City is a forty-minute drive. In spite of the upscale reputation of that part of town, the hospital itself is a shabby clinic in a tattered building. Mom and Dad are doubtless taken aback. This isn't what they expected. They check Richard in and are told to wait in a dim-lit reception area amid the harsh acoustics and sour smells of an understaffed urban hospital. After a short wait a doctor addresses the threesome and explains in nebulous detail what they have in store for

Richard. A tube (catheter) will be inserted into the femoral artery at the groin and threaded up into the right side of the heart where they plan to take pressure readings, along with a few pictures. It all sounds strange enough, and everyone, Richard included, appears a little startled. A radio-opaque dye will be injected into the heart that will show up on an X ray. A miracle of modern science. An angiogram, they call it. Ingenious.

Richard says goodbye to Mom and Dad with a brief hug, and leaves with the doctor down a dark corridor to a private room where he is asked to disrobe. The doctor tells him a male nurse will be in shortly to prep him for the procedure, then leaves through an oak door holding a translucent pane of sanded glass. Richard strips in the sudden quiet down to his underwear, and waits in the slight chill and muddled sounds of the hospital on a table covered with starched rice paper. Soon the door swings open and a man with a clipboard and white jacket steps in.

Richard does what he asks. He is suddenly afraid of what is about to happen. The nurse has him lie back, naked, beneath a large electric light. He slits his eyes against the brightness. Suddenly he feels the two hands and the cool steel blade as it mows a path through the pubic hair around his groin. He is shocked. Tears rise up in his eyes. He feels his throat harden as he peers down over his chest at what's happening to him. Eventually he is asked to relax by the anonymous voice beyond his field of view. He tries and manages to do so. Then he closes his eyes against it all.

Mom, Dad and the doctor are conferring at the reception desk the following day when Richard finally reappears. They both hug him, feeling the deep tremors of his body, and ask how he feels.

"All right," he says, giving away no details. He now feels he harbors a humiliation.

The doctor eventually appears and tells Mom and Dad how they had a little trouble with the cylinder of radio-opaque dye, which produced a delay, but that Richard had behaved brilliantly. He remarks about his courage and stoicism. The doctor explains that they would like to do a few more noninvasive tests the following day, and then they will have a clear idea of what's wrong with Richard's heart.

When I see him later in the week he is strangely quiet and reclusive. "Still can't play basketball," he mutters from behind the curtain of a broad book as he lies reposed upon his bed. And that is all I will learn about it for years to come. Richard now has, and always will have in my imagination, a face that doesn't match his years. It is the face of a ruined child.

8

Newark Academy is a rich all-boys school in the gutted heart of the city that offers a more rigorous academic milieu than the public schools. As a thirteen-year-old I assimilate myself into a coterie of five friends: two Jews, a German Catholic and two Italians. A peculiar conglomeration. As one of the two Jews I am the webby tissue that binds us into a cloister. Our secular social dynamics are dictated by the two basic laws of nature and society: gravity and inertia; Judaism and Catholicism. Last year I was bar-mitzvahed and am now viewed as a man through the lens of my faith.

We have mysterious relations with one another. John Ritota, an Italian friend, is one of many wealthy paisan families who send their children to the academy. Theirs is an exclusive clique. They are uninhibited in their public displays of affection toward one another, yet keep outsiders at arm's length in subtle and uniquely Italian ways.

Jews are a similar breed. Perhaps it is a nature common to races sprung from the Mediterranean. Of course exceptions in the temperament of family relations exist; both my and my friend Marty's families are customarily more formal. Marty's father is a Russian Jew who came to America by way of the Orient just prior to World War II. The family history carries with it the force of myth, with the strange mixture of Asian aristocracy, the ancient grandeur of Czarist Russia. His father's peculiar accent and dress suggest a foreign demeanor of regal proportions in keeping with the palatial family home. Though his son Marty is very intelligent, he is not adequately motivated for genius, as his father seems to expect. In the glare of his father's eyes, I am, as a friend, an accessory to Marty's relative lack of ambition, a co-conspirator with three Catholics.

With haunting clarity, I now see deep in my mind's eye the Newark Academy building itself as a reflection of our con-glomerated relations, a decaying anachronism at the epicenter of a shattered American city. The girth of its arched roof beam is intended to impress, as are the marble pillars standing like petri-fied forelegs of Asian elephants at the summit of the stairs. On all sides it is surrounded by urban dry-rot, flaking brick, the va-cant eyes of central Newark residents, the Doppler howl of a passing ambulance, the blue glitter of crushed glass sparkling in shadows between mortifying attempts at urban renewal. With my friends I feel a precious equilibrium, a focus developing, maturation. Within our group the mythical past stands leavened by the-way-it-is, a phenomenon born of an ever-widening gap in generational sensibilities. No one could be happier among these ruins.

9

The following fall Richard must have gone to Dr. Gillette for another checkup, because suddenly it has been arranged for us both to go to the National Institutes of Health in Bethesda, Maryland. The event is grandiose. It is also entirely unexpected that our matching hearts could draw such interest. Years later I will learn Gillette has recently read an article on a disease that has until now been poorly described, called Idiopathic Hypertrophic Subaortic Stenosis, or IHSS. The article was written by an old medical school friend by the name of Eugene Braunwald, a man who will one day become perhaps the most widely renowned cardiologist in the United States. Gillette apparently thinks the disease described in this article has something to do with Richard's illness and our mother's death. Braunwald agrees and has invited us both down to the NIH for a full week in the fall.

Not until we arrive do we have any idea what the NIH is about. As the new Continental convertible rolls past building after building of what appears to be part of a whole by virtue of its sameness, we come upon a brick sign built into a neat lawn: WELCOME TO THE NATIONAL INSTITUTES OF HEALTH. Dad holds his directions in one hand while recklessly steering with the other. He tells us all to be on the lookout for Building 10. The place has the vast layout of a university campus, so it takes a bit of driving around to find it. Dad points out that across the street is the U.S. Naval Hospital where the President is cared for. This is also where Kennedy's body was taken after being shot in Dallas the year before last. Finally we locate the building, park the Continental in a distant lot and together we make the hike to check in.

From the beginning the Institutes overwhelm. Entire floors appear to be dedicated to specific diseases and organs. As we arrived I noticed the various departments: oncology, hepatology, nephrology, pulmonary and cardiology, which is where we are now. Though very few people are aware of it, the NIH is entirely funded by the government, and any federal money appropriated for health care is first allocated through the NIH. The only way you can get admitted is to have a disease they are studying at the time. All your medical care is free, but first you must sign document after document stating that you understand this is a research hospital, that you'll be given treatment the efficacy of which has yet to be proven. This takes away the burden of responsibility from them if anything happens to you. It is made clear you are a white rat, but a very well-cared-for white rat. This is an assembly of some of the greatest medical minds in the world, and their attention is focused on *you*.

When we check in the receptionist hands us each an itinerary of what they have planned for us. The last procedure will be a right and left heart catheterization. Just as Richard expected. After that we're home free, since all other procedures are noninvasive. But there it stands like a monolith.

Eventually the chief of cardiology for the entire NIH, Dr. Braunwald, introduces himself to Mom and Dad, then to Richard and me. He is a very large, very imposing and serious man, someone who obviously operates with natural ease in a sterile academic setting. From the very beginning I have learned to associate cardiologists with social misfits, and perhaps this stereotype has sprouted in my mind with this initial introduction to

Dr. Braunwald. He does not come across as a warm man. But he is brilliant, and this has been made very clear, first by Dr. Gillette, then by Dad.

While Braunwald expounds upon what he has planned for us, Dad interrupts him during a caesura in his speech and points out that Richard has already had a heart catheterization, the results of which are at Flower Fifth Hospital in New York. Couldn't they simply call up there for the findings?

Braunwald is wagging his head before Dad finishes his sentence to show his disinterest in their data. With that single gesture he tells us everything done for Richard heretofore has been foolishness. He wearily cites their expertise, that they don't trust anyone else's findings. It must be done again. That settles it for our parents.

Richard and I hug Mom and Dad, say goodbye, then we're led away by a nurse. The moment we arrive on the ward a whole team of doctors and nurses greets us as though we are lost family. Almost immediately Richard asks about the catheterization, if what they plan to do is the same as what was done at Flower Fifth. He quickly begins describing the procedure in simplistic terms, and another nurse replies, "Yep, that's pretty much a heart cath."

The first two days are a walk through the garden, the procedures being all noninvasive. Without the immediate prospect of pain the beginning of the week becomes adventurous. Electrocardiograms are taken, treadmill tests given, all in a spirit of celebration. Even Richard's spirits lighten; he makes incredibly witty jokes and lays on the charm in a way I never can.

But after the two days of noninvasive testing is completed, Richard is prepped and cathed. When he comes off the table two hours later he is trembling a bit, but by-and-large is okay. "This is no Flower Fifth," he remarks. The procedure was done quickly, competently. The staff is the best in the world. Clearly there is a certain pride among them connected to the Institutes' reputation.

Then it is my turn. As I am lying back on the table, a cardiologist says, "Okay, Bobby. You're going to feel a little needle stick in your groin where my fingers are. It'll hurt like you're at the dentist." This is my first introduction to the world of clinical medicine.

In contrast to Richard's restraint throughout our stay, I wallow in the attention, making jokes, flirting with the nurses. Having this many people paying attention to me is a high. I want them to be in awe, to be struck by my courage and threshold of pain. Considering the circumstances the fantasy is a little sick. These people plan to run a plastic tube through my veins and arteries to uncover the secrets of a fourteen-year-old heart. Nevertheless, the surgical table becomes a stage.

A tremendous pressure fills the groin as an immense and bony palm presses against the femoral artery. Then I feel a pop. They have entered the artery. The only relief I know in the lab is this anonymous black hand, and these two brown eyes. After a few minutes I feel the catheter turn down into the aorta and slither into my heart. Every now and then it skips a beat when the plastic catheter touches the inner walls of the chambers. The jokes stop, and I squeeze the warm black flesh.

"You're scaring me," I say to the nurse. "My heart's skipping."

The cardiologist raises his head. I see the crown of his blue surgical cap rise up and hear him say from behind the mask, "You'll be all right. That's normal."

When they are ready to inject the dye, the cardiologist's head appears again to tell me what to expect. I will feel extremely nauseated for about thirty seconds, and an intense heat will emanate from my chest. That's the body's reaction to the dye; again, these sensations are normal.

Heat surges down my chest and centers itself in my groin, but once the angiogram is complete the cardiologist explains that they are now going to give me a drug that will provoke obstruction of bloodflow out of the heart, reproducing the dizzy spells that Richard experienced when playing basketball. The drug is amyl nitrate, what will come to be known on the street as *poppers* for recreational use toward the end of the decade.

Another nurse breaks a capsule under my nose and instructs me to inhale. Suddenly I feel my heart sprint in my chest. I now think I am about to die, that they really do want to burst my heart. My face flushes with the sudden rush of new blood followed by an abrupt dearth once the obstruction is formed. The heart pounds as though it were sentient, and is now scared absolutely senseless. Then, as quickly as the effect of the popper appeared, it vanishes in a fog. The tests are complete for the day, the data has been culled. Now there are only voices of praise for having endured this brief terror without whining. Once again I realize I am the center of attention and bask in the artificial glory of not having snapped under the weight of fear. The nurse squeezes my moist hand.

That day Richard and I are laid up in bed together in the same room with sandbags over our groins to keep direct pressure on our matching wounds. This is the source of a string of lewd jokes I accost the nurses with each time they enter our room. But Richard remains subdued, his mind seemingly elsewhere. He loses himself in books, his fingernails curled against his teeth behind the pages. Every now and then when he emerges to eat or relieve himself, he remains distant, seemingly content in a mood of melancholy.

Toward the end of the week Dr. Braunwald along with a couple of other staff cardiologists gather Mom, Dad, Richard and myself at the foot of our bed. The testing is complete, and Braunwald is prepared with the bottom line on Richard's condition and my future. Again, he appears ominously serious, but not grave. He's simply a serious man and can't help but invest a discussion with an air of solemnity. Dad's brow pinches as he listens, bobbing his head from time to time, and asks questions. Mom murmurs general agreement and understanding. Richard and I listen peripherally in silence.

The bottom line, as Braunwald puts it, is that Richard definitely has IHSS, the rare disease he has recently written about. Sudden death is possible if he were to take up basketball again, so it will remain forbidden. Not much is known about the disease, he continues, but it is something like having a muscle-bound heart. When exercising vigorously the heart walls thicken like any other muscle, and the chambers cannot fill or empty to normal capacity. That's what causes the dizzy spells on the court. If Richard continues to play, his heart could begin beating arrhythmically, merely jiggling like a can of worms instead of with a coordinated rhythm that moves the blood efficiently. If that happens it could be life-threatening and death may be sudden.* I, on the other hand, do not have the disease. Not yet, anyway. But they want to watch me. Each year I will be scheduled in for tests along with Richard. I interpret this message as being let off the hook.

---

*Ideopathic Hypertrophic Subaortic Stenosis (IHSS) is now called Hypertrophic Cardiomyopathy (HCM). It is usually a genetically inherited, slowly progressive disease of the muscle of the heart which causes thickening of the walls, obstructing blood flow into and out of the chambers. Stiffening of the heart's walls usually develops, which in turn leads to severe shortness of breath and, ultimately, heart failure. The disease is the leading cause of sudden death among young athletes. Former Loyola Marymount basketball All-American Hank Gathers dropped dead on the court in his senior year of college after having been diagnosed with HCM. It was also recently debated whether or not former Boston Celtic Captain Reggie Lewis also died from this same disease.

10

Richard dates a Catholic girl, Linda Kelley, whom our mother forbids him to see. I observe the exchanges of rage and misunderstanding from the shadows and emptiness of other rooms. And for my part I've been making weekend forays to Greenwich Village. It is a bawdy business I love, rambling through the fetid congested throng against the lazy sounds of jazz ushering out of darkened doorways leading into dimly lit rooms layered with yellow smoke. On the first of these journeys I wear Top-Siders and my blue academy blazer, not having been home yet from school. I naively make my way through the alternating images of swank and squalor with disciplined vigilance, looking like a friend of Howdy Doody's who got off on the wrong exit. But I'm on it, I'm cool. After a few trips, the clothes change, the hair goes without a cut. I now walk the walk. In the meantime my parents are thoroughly bewildered. As a half-measure of retaliation and a half of correction, our mother decides we are to become observant Jews. The decision is intended either to rein in or alienate Richard, as observant Jews traditionally date other observant Jews exclusively. Of course it fails in the former and succeeds in the latter. To Mom, my behavior is an auxiliary problem. Unhappy families are unhappy in their own way, and ours has grown uniquely miserable.

But unseen forces are at work. As Richard and I have changed, so have all families, neighborhoods and cities. It is 1965. Greenwich Village is the seminal turf of modern American culture, the center of the universe. At age fifteen I step off the bus every Friday, onto the crumbling mortar and gravel conglomeration running along the streets. I look down the tall dark corridor of flop buildings where the funky rhythms of jazz pour through metal grates over windows. Everywhere is the unanimous soft thump of a wide drum, a clarinet and cornet before black cheeks bloated with air, thrusting breath through brass valves, driven up to the proper key and held there with infinite patience. The dingy primary colors of billboards stand over sidewalks glittering with slivers and cusps of broken glass. Every weekend I walk past the vulgar propositions of prostitutes standing in the shadows of doorways to the panel houses above with my small group of friends.

But the decade evolves and mutates. The summer of 1967 is hot. From the beginning of spring it is as though the world has tilted, taking sunlight at a more obtuse angle. Something seems to have snapped across the Republic, a malaise afflicting the citizenry. The people are scared of one another, and Walter Cronkite demonstrates this nightly.

On the blue flickering television in our living room I watch the police who wear World War I–style helmets as they stand before a burning car during the Newark race riots. A fire engine arrives on the scene and is pelted with chunks of concrete. The police disperse, being unprepared for this, and scatter throughout the city.

Each night on the television images of burning buildings, looters, and National Guard troops fill the screen within the haze of tear gas. It taxes the imagination that all this is occurring just eight or ten miles from home. Yet the suburbs of Newark remain untouched, like an infant in an incubator. All across the nation riots erupt in Watts, Detroit and Cleveland. The roof has been torn from the Republic. The apocalypse is forecast and expected to be televised, brought to our living room in living color.

When the riots have finally run their course a few days later, twenty-three people are dead: a white fireman, a white detective and twenty-one blacks. Six are women, two are children.

Toward the end of the week absentee workers begin appearing at my father's factory at 8:00 A.M., ready to work. They have the wild reckless look of spiritual abandonment in their eye. They haven't slept for days, yet they are fully awake, fully alive. Eyes are moist and bloodshot, their dress flamboyantly haphazard. There is the distinct air about them that they don't give a damn anymore.

At seventeen I cannot condone the riots, but I understand these people, the latent anger they carry in their hearts as they move about a white world, and the violent expression of it with the introduction of hopelessness.

During these times I only see Richard from time to time when he stops by the house while no one is home. He pulls up the neat slab of asphalt driveway in an old Buick with faded red and black paint. He is angry and brilliant and alone, with only Linda and a few close male friends. Two years ago he graduated from high school as a National Merit Scholar, and was accepted into medical school at age eighteen, but it is now unclear whether or not he has the desire to get through. I see the shadow of terror in the whites of his eyes as they swim in an obscure haze when we talk. Though he admits to no fear, no loneliness, it shows in the amplified nervousness of his every gesture.

At night images come to me with the force of nightmare: the pale skin drawn tight about his skull, the quiet terror lying just below the glassy pools of his eyes, the mounting fatigue in his gait as the invisible illness comes to bear. Right now I imagine him frenetically roaming the city in that old Buick with a lot of improperly turned ideas rising within the vault of his mind, his sick and nervous heart, running on clean adrenaline, providing a gas-blue flame.

It is the company of others that goes furthest toward erasing everyday terrors. This is my unconscious belief. The terror to which the ordinary madman is attuned, the resolution of physical reality magnified beyond comprehension—there lies the pith of loneliness. When the world within the silent vault of consciousness can no longer be reconciled with outside phenomena, the bedrock of loneliness is revealed. Other human beings are the receptors of communication, windows between worlds. Without them isolation is absolute, and isolation is the germ of all madness.

THE HORSE

II

Boulder, Colorado, 1968: the salmon pink of sandstone, a dirty sky welded to an arc of wildgrass, stones sunk into the ground over the ancient graves of dinosaurs. A university built of flagstone on a hill.

Before deciding upon a college last year I saw the red and pink dirt, the peculiar architecture and lush deciduous trees on a brochure I had requested from the University of Colorado. I wanted to get away as soon as and as far as I could from Livingston, and Boulder was geographically and culturally distant. I saw the town was somehow congruent with the changing times, fashionable in an esoteric way, and decided to matriculate there based on these impressions.

But it was ten weeks from graduation day at Newark Academy until classes began in Boulder. I came up with the pretext to leave for my Uncle Bill and Aunt Janice's home in Los Angeles with plans of taking an introductory class in chemistry at the local community college, so the departure would have the blessing of Mom and Dad. Within days of graduation I was flying west.

Now, as the plane descends into the thin brown cloud, I scan the horizon of the Pacific Ocean. I imagine the Orient, the Pacific Rim, names such as Guam, Beijing, Burma, and suddenly feel a very long way from home. The vast blue desert quickly fades into a sea of concrete as the plane lowers into the city. The fuselage shudders, the tires shriek against the earth. As the plane slows coming off the tarmac and I gaze about the neo-modern of LAX, the space-age look of the airport itself, and tell myself what an immense world this is.

My aunt and uncle offer home and stability, which I need and abruptly shun whenever the spirit moves me. And the spirit moves me nearly every day. I am eighteen and free for the first time in my life. I buy a battered red Cutlass convertible with money earned working at my father's factory. At night I cruise up the moonlit coast on Highway One, or take an occasional trip to Sunset Boulevard to mingle among the pimps and prostitutes, try to come to know the city at its most grisly, personal level. In my aunt and uncle's home I possess the status of neither adolescent nor adult, so during the long languid days I come to know my three young cousins. The youngest, Jeff, is seven, his older brother Jon is ten. Jessica, the oldest, is twelve and burdened with severe juvenile diabetes.

The summer is hot, dry, bright and unremarkable except for the ocular clarity of a singular memory. Jessica sits on the ivory lid of a toilet at home, her summer dress hiked up to her small right hip. With one hand she digs into the shiny worn pocket of the dress and produces a vial of insulin and a syringe. She adroitly pops the plastic cap off, exposing the fresh needle, and sinks it into the rubber belly of the upturned vial. She carefully and quickly draws the plunger from the plastic cylinder, and the chamber fills. Then, within the same motion, she points the needle skyward, taps the air bubbles to the top, and thrusts a jet of liquid onto the bathroom tile. A moment later she jabs the needle into her exposed thigh, giving away but a faint wince, an involuntary twitch of young musculature. The plunger is compressed, the needle withdrawn, her skirt thrown down, and she bolts past me out the door to friends outside playing a game of hopscotch on the sidewalk. I see on the bathroom countertop that she has forgotten her stick of pastel chalk and a smooth stone. I pick them up and take them out to her where she has already involved herself in the game.

At twelve she is insulin-dependent. Without it she will die, and she knows this. She carries a vial, hypodermic needle and a candy bar on her person wherever she goes. She knows how to adjust her insulin doses, having given herself injections since age five. She doesn't slow down unless feeling hypoglycemic, in which case she nibbles at the candy bar until her spirit returns like a ghost suddenly possessing her body. She is gentle, precocious and in command of a towering intellect.

One afternoon I take all three of my cousins to an antiwar demonstration in the convertible. As we drive into downtown L.A. the traffic grows thick with Volkswagens and beat-up cars filled with sweaty college students dressed in rather gamy-looking jeans and T-shirts. Jessica rides shotgun. When I point out that we must be getting near, she asks why protesters tend to dress the way they do.

"They don't like the world the way it is," I say at a loss for anything more insightful.

"Anything about it?"

"At least the way adults dress."

The wind twirls her dark hair into her eyes, and she gently brushes it away.

Through the years diabetes will ravage her organs. I will glimpse her struggle for life in piecemeal fashion from a distance, but from a unique vantage. All I can say is that for her it is a blessing the world was made round. That way she cannot see what lies just over the horizon.

I have touched down on another planet. Boulder is so unfamiliar, so exotic and surreal, the very ground is of a different color, the semiarid foothills, the Martian-like sunsets, the pink and orange sky at dusk.

I move into a dormitory that first year and make friends with a small coterie of sullen Marxist intellectuals and flamboyant political activists. They would be academic clichés were it not for their ardor. Each week we attend Students for a Democratic Society meetings at the student union. Political discussions, driven by amphetamines and caffeine, mill into the small hours of dawn, while elsewhere on campus much of the same carries on. Politics and political philosophy are fashionable. The campus and town are caught up in the cool frenzy of revolution, each day possessing the unnameable but palpable quality that history is being produced locally.

SDS meetings present speakers from the Black Student Alliance, the Weathermen—before their notorious terrorist activities in Madison and Berkeley—and the Black Panthers. Voices of keynote speakers fill the stone auditorium with an uninhibited rage, the likes of which I've never seen. They are brilliant and angry. There is a precision to their rancor, a sophistication in the language they employ that convinces with its delicate tenacity. It is their audacity that astounds, as they themselves seldom obey the very logic they impose on others.

The landscape of these days has about them the air that something is about to happen, that anything might happen. I am dizzy with astonishment. The gentle pace of undergraduate academia affords time to contemplate the world beyond the bubble of university life. And there is much to contemplate, as the Nixon Administration busies itself with escalating the Vietnam war. Or such is the Zeitgeist among students at least, certainly among SDS members. The organization commits considerable resources to organizing antiwar demonstrations across the west, and tacitly inciting mayhem within the bureaucracy of the University of Colorado itself. It is suspected the university holds

stock in Dow Chemical Corporation, the manufacturer of na-
palm and other war matériel. It is 1968.

One day in the early fall, a day I recall for the fine gray rain
falling on my way to the university, I arrive late at my math class
wet, cold and out of breath. I collapse into the small wooden
desk, ignoring the attention I've drawn to myself. The class rustles a moment as everyone turns and gawks. I wipe away droplets
from my brow, dry off my glasses, and carefully slide them on
with a forefinger against the bridge. My vision is foggy with
warm condensation lifting from my face and collecting on the
cold lenses. Once the vapor drifts from the glass, I see a face staring at me, the eyes smiling.

All through math class, while the professor walks to and fro
before the blackboard with a slender cylinder of white chalk in
his hand, my mind stutters with fascination. Her auburn hair is
fashionably long and doll-like. I stare at the hourglass shape of
the back of her head as it drifts left and right, following the professor's pendulous motion. The corner of her mouth holds the
same grimace. I see the smooth skin drawn up into the cheek,
the crease of the eye cutting into the temple.

After class I pause outside the door, ostensibly to adjust the
leather strap of my backpack. In my corner vision I see her approach with the same shy smile, a slightly lowered forehead
meant to conceal the mouth. She can't help but smile at me, I
tell myself, and my heart surges.

We weave our way through a wet stream of students down the
long tall hallway to a pair of doors. Outside an infinitely fine rain
is drizzling over the red slate rooftops of campus. I ask if she
would like to go for a cup of coffee at the union. She nods, neither looking me in the eye nor saying anything. Just a simple,
decisive nod as she gazes straight ahead through slit eyes, her
mouth shaped into a slight grin.

We sit at a square table across from one another amid the

clamor of students rushing to class. A pale wreath of steam lifts from the surface of dark coffee and disappears against her innocent face. We sit, neither of us attempting to speak against the noise until the rush has passed. Then she tells me about herself: Ann, a Protestant girl from Oregon, daughter of a lawyer. Concerned with the Administration's policy in Southeast Asia. She doesn't wear makeup. Her natural beauty is what attracts me to her. She is very reserved, and shows hints of the existential pain I have come to identify with. I feel at ease and am drawn to her as a moth to light.

12

That first fall I feel the dramatic effects of the tiny war within my heart. For the first time I experience the momentary terror of having my life threatened when playing basketball. Dizzy spells strike with a fury, producing a sense of utter vertigo. When this occurs on public courts in Boulder, I drop my head between my knees, flooding my skull with fresh blood, and the threat vanishes. But within just a few weeks the symptoms become noticeably more acute. When I call the NIH to talk with Dr. Epstein, the new chief of cardiology who has replaced Dr. Braunwald, he tells me I don't appreciate the life-threatening nature of the symptoms. I could drop dead on the court, so it's imperative that I not play. He also wants to see me, and promises plane tickets. An appointment is made for the following week, and so the routine of school is severed just two months after it starts. I abruptly leave town, giving away few details to new friends, with the exception of Ann, of the fears that I harbor.

I fly out of Stapleton Airport in Denver in the middle of the night, leaving behind the hubbub of Boulder. It is a peculiar flight, in many ways my first night as an adult. The plane is nearly empty but for a young family huddled toward the back of the fuselage. I am alone and on my way to a hospital. During the four-hour flight I gaze through an oval window at the eerie gray light illuminating the tops of small dense clouds. The wrinkled pillows stand over the midwest like the cerebrums of giants as I soar over within the isolated hum of the pressurized cabin. To me the flight represents the silent and lonely transition between the world of hospitals and the world of the living. I feel the continent beneath me, North America. I sense the gravity of these days.

At NIH I am again told of what lies in store for me: a right and left heart catheterization is scheduled, and suddenly I don't feel up to all this by myself. Richard isn't here to share and deflect the strangeness and pain; Mom and Dad won't be down until after the invasive procedures are completed. I need family here and now, I need Ann.

The following morning I'm reintroduced to the vaguely familiar men and women of the cath lab. My body is prepped and bathed in disinfectant, then hauled to the operating table at the center of the room. I grow convivial as the anxiety builds. The doctors prepare needles of local anesthetic, pointing the glinting spires at threatening trajectories. A phony conversation picks up with questions concerning Boulder and my chosen field of study there. I tell them I want to be a doctor, and hearing this pleases them immensely. They begin explaining what they're about to do as though I already were a medical student. I am charmed through flattery; anxiety is vaporized. I play the role of the distinguished observer-patient-physician and eager student as needles of anesthesia float toward me. I become detached from this body as I repress my own reactive fear and replace it with deigned fascination. I ask for a mirror to see what is taking place at the crease of both elbows and proceed to intellectualize the small bloody scenes as if they were part of someone else. As the tubes are inserted I am no longer the victim of what lies before my eyes in the rectangle of mirror, but the curious unattached observer.

The catheters swim into my heart, pressures are taken, a green dye is injected. Then I am asked to stand up, walk to the treadmill with these tubes protruding from my arms to see how my pressures are affected when I exercise. Initially I keep my fear in check because their attitude about actually having me do this seems routine. But this is an experiment. I remain quiet as they confer among themselves.

So with tubes inserted into my heart, I sit up, waddle to the treadmill lab down the hall, and work out. My heart skips every now and then as the plastic touches the chamber walls. In the lower corners of my vision I watch the clear tubes of green dye rush into the labyrinth of my body. A question rises up, slowly and subtly, from an obscure recess of consciousness. At this moment the question is a secret to me, released like a gas bubble from the muddy bottom of a pond wiggling its way toward the surface: Do these people really love me?

I3

Dr. Epstein stands at the foot of the bed, his face and gestures expressionless. With stupefying candor he tells me I have IHSS, the disease my brother has, the disease my mother most likely died of. Within the same sentence he digresses into a jargon-riddled explanation of why and how they know.

Mom and Dad are here, bedside, revising and couching the news so that it doesn't overwhelm. I am uninterested, a little numb, but not from shock or fear. I have long suspected this. Knowing and suspicion have undergone a process of alchemy to become a sort of unconscious certainty. He tells me I will need a cardiologist in Colorado to monitor the heart. At the University of Colorado Hospital in Denver is a man by the name of Dr. Gil Blount whom I am to look up upon my return to Boulder. Sports of course are forbidden. He goes on to prescribe the drug Inderal to decrease the severity of the dizzy spells. Inderal is a beta blocker, he tells us—a drug that lessens the effect of adrenaline on the nervous system. This will keep the heart from responding too vigorously to simple daily thrills. The drug has some side effects, including decrease in sex drive and depression. In small ways the rapture of what it means to be alive may wash out of my daily life. But it is a mild dose, he says. Then he leaves.

Later that day I am discharged. I have to be getting back to Boulder. On the way to the airport I tell Mom and Dad about school. The conversation is a heavily edited briefing, details being innocuous and general. I say goodbye with a bland sort of reluctance. I see myself as an adult, a big boy, and am passively resentful of their parental impulses. I have recently learned their marriage is on the rocks, which, I must admit, neither pleases nor displeases me. Certainly it doesn't surprise me. We exchange modest hugs, and once again I am soaring over the craton of North America, into this strange small town of red and blond rock that lies against the foothills of the Rockies.

Back in Boulder I decide I am getting sick because I am overweight. The idea is contrary to the science of cardiology, which I am coming to admire in a personal, obsessive way, but I am certain of it. I buy a rubber suit, something a boxer might use to shed water weight before a fight. At dusk I leave the flagstone dormitory for the university basketball courts. Once the sun slips behind the silhouette of mountains, the dry mountain air quickly cools, sunlight dies abruptly in an orange and red haze that lingers, submerging the streets in shadows. Dusk is a magical time, a phenomenon unknown in the east. The cool and darkening atmosphere invigorates the town.

At the basketball court I dribble a ball back and forth, feeling the sweat condense within the soft cotton T-shirt beneath the rubber second skin. Blood-warm streams leak steadily from the ankles and pool in my shoes. The rubber squeaks with wetness at the joints; my mind swims, it seems, in a cloud of vapor. The colorful evening shades of Boulder at dusk, and the ethereal effect of dizziness create a dreamscape. For a short time I am removed from this body, high above it all. I can overcome disease through sheer tenacity, controlled direction of will. The cadence of the ball against the concrete mixes with the throbbing of my heart, stream of consciousness takes over, and I become brilliant, invincible, immune to pain and worry. IHSS is a rumor believed by the lazy. I vow to wring this disease from my body like sweat.

But the following month the dizzy spells grow more severe. I call Richard in California from time to time, generally when loneliness intrudes on the day. The immediate sharing of experience brings quick though temporary relief. He is sick and certainly getting worse, no doubt about it. But the phone calls are brief. He gets manic, the volume and tone of his voice flutter beyond control. He and Linda are now married, so we talk about that for a while. But always there is the disease, and somehow the topic insidiously finds its way back to the center. This is my older brother, the man whom I am tied to in mind and body, a vague reflection of myself. He is someone I both fear and admire. Apart from Ann, there really is no one else with whom I share what this life has been like.

One day I call the NIH and talk to Dr. Epstein about the symptoms intensifying in spite of the Inderal. He asks if I've contacted Dr. Blount, and I tell him I haven't yet. From that point on his voice conveys resignation at my lackadaisical attitude. I still don't appreciate the life-threatening aspects of IHSS. That's all he has to say.

So sometime in late fall I call Dr. Blount's office. He speaks enthusiastically and optimistically over the phone. He says he has been waiting for my call. He knows of my illness, and says that I should visit him soon. I don't mention the silent and desperate gloominess that has settled over my first semester at school, how I've witnessed the colors wash out of the town with the approach of winter. Perhaps it is part of the initial effects of the Inderal, yet I can't imagine everyday life without the dour imagery I now superimpose upon every scene I come upon.

The hospital, the University of Colorado Health Science Center, stands to the side of a corridor with a throng of cars, students, doctors and medical staff pulsing through a canyon of buildings. There is a distinct academic air here, even in the street, a professional grubbiness that makes me feel not so very far from Boulder. The red brick of the Denver V.A. hospital is just down the street, adding to the slow-moving traffic and the weightiness of the times. The seemingly windowless building holds special significance in 1968.

After a short search I find Dr. Blount's office deep within the hospital. I knock on his door, and a voice promptly invites me in. A man with straight silver hair smoothed against his skull turns in a wooden swivel chair and smiles.

"You must be Bob Pensack." His voice is commanding. "Come in, come in."

When he stands I see he is tall and thin, and for a man in his late fifties, somewhat eccentric in his dress. I imagine him as an English gentleman, as he wears his hair long and tapered against the slender nape of his neck, a style more in keeping with conventional taste over there than here. His voice carries a New England accent, with its observance of obscure propriety and exotic taste. About his neck is strung a Leatham stethoscope, the finest and most sensitive in the world. The only other place I've seen a Leatham stethoscope, which is British also, is at the NIH. I already know that only real cardiologists have any use for them. A warm and powerful man, a voice that makes me feel safe. In his shadow the disease of IHSS looks paltry. I imagine he understands the mysterious operations of the heart with the heightened sense of intuition, that he has the transcendent knowledge of cardiology as art and craft, not mere science. These are my first and lasting impressions.

Dr. Blount has me sit on a small stool and pull off my shirt. He lowers the finely fluted steel of the stethoscope over his head and places a hand on my naked back. With the other he holds the sensor to my chest and coasts it over the contours in a delicate pattern. I notice his breathing is irregular; he controls the rhythm so as to create moments of silence, a vacuum filled by the report of this strange young heart in his ears. I feel the wind of his breath against my skin and wonder what he's hearing between each draw. The next time he speaks, I am thinking, he will tell me how to fix this heart, for my confidence in this man is absolute. After several expanded minutes he exhales through his nostrils, pulls the Leatham from his ears and drapes it over his shoulders.

"Well." He pauses for effect and sets his palms onto his large bony knees. "There's clearly a murmur."

"The dizzy spells have gotten worse," I say.

"Have you been taking the Inderal?"

"Yeah."

"Has it helped?"

"Not that I can tell."

"I'll need to talk with Dr. Epstein in Maryland about this." He rotates about in his swivel chair, then searches through his Rolodex for Epstein's number. It takes a few minutes for the call to get through, but once it does the conversation is brief and decisive. After hanging up, Dr. Blount reiterates what I heard him agree to over the phone. My Inderal prescription will be roughly doubled, which will hopefully keep the heart from obstructing so severely. The side effects of depression and listlessness are expected to become more prominent. He smiles plaintively. His large hands encompass his kneecaps, his eyes display real compassion.

"This is all I can do for now, young man. If the side effects become too obtrusive, call me right away."

A string of ruby taillights drifts over the shallow hills of prairie on the drive back to Boulder. Darkness encases the car as the sun sinks further and further behind the mountains. I turn on the A.M. radio and roll the dial across the warbling frequencies, static and cosmic squeal that dominate the speaker. Nothing comes in clearly, not even the inane pop music stations. I flick the radio off and sit within the hum of the motor and howl of the wind for a moment, then roll down the window. The jet of cold air attacks the ears, refreshes the mind. Soon the silver and gold lights of Boulder glitter at the bottom of a vast draw. For a moment I pull the car out of gear and allow it to run down the steepening grade. The wind rages in my ears, the car shimmies as the white needle glides across the speedometer dial. Taillights rush past and grow bleary through my moistened vision, and I momentarily lose myself in the momentum of the runaway car. There is nothing to be done, I tell myself. Nothing at all.

Once into the routine of school, the days stack neatly into months. Every morning I sling a canvas backpack filled with notebooks and textbooks over my shoulder, then leave the flagstone dormitory by way of a short wooden door, and walk through a barren winter garden to the university. Each morning I find birds singing madly within a maple tree, then cease as I pass below. The sudden silence inexplicably terrifies me. My breath is a gentle pant when I arrive at class. Through the bright winter months my days become a routine void of the familiar flashes of condensed life that keep depression from consuming the mind. Melancholy descends like a veil, turning grim thoughts inward.

14

By springtime Ann and I are intimates. As our freshman year progresses, our dependence on one another declares itself. We study together, dream together, and learn from one another. But an unsettling pattern develops in our relations: each afternoon we spend together in agonizing Platonic love on a make-believe date; then as night falls, she often grows restless and makes excuses to leave in the midst of a good time.

Incrementally our relationship evolves into an affair. Moist hands occasionally tremble against an upper thigh. The unsteady hand is pushed away, but it returns again and again, relentlessly, until there is a release of some sort. Always we are on the verge of brave moments.

We are now sitting at an outdoor café. It is August, summer school has ended, the town emptied in the transition, and Ann has just returned from summer break in Oregon. Her skin has tanned evenly through the summer months, and now has a wonderful burnished quality about it. The color of sandstone. Sunglasses hide her eyes.

She looks off toward the plains, then lifts her face to the potent sun. She swipes at her brown beer bottle and recklessly lays the mouth upon her lower lip and swallows hard. I let a moment of silence fall between us as I observe the bronze column of cartilage rhythmically gesticulating within her strong neck. Eventually she sets the voided bottle down on the metal tabletop and cocks her head to take the sunlight more evenly.

As we sit in awkward silence at the table, I can tell she is antsy. I watch her stare off into the plains; she is about to make one of her abrupt departures, which of course makes me anxious.

"I'm living in that basement apartment on College Avenue," I say to jar her thoughts. "I want you to forget about the sorority house and move in with me."

She is silent for a moment, then her head begins to nod, gently at first, then more decisively. "It's just a couple of blocks away, right?"

"Three blocks. I have the key with me."

We walk together down the ragged sidewalk, past the hippies, the speed freaks, the fanatics declaring manifestos. Just a block beyond all the madness the house rises up within a wild lawn of chokecherries, waist-high spears of prairie grass and rosebushes. Nothing terribly uncommon for a liberal arts college town, but peculiar by any standard. I lead Ann by the hand over the river rock path obscured by overgrown flora to the basement door, then jimmy the key around in the old brass lock for some time before the dead bolt slides clear and the door gives way to a dank darkness.

The house is cavernous, the exposed pipes are painted in flamboyant colors. Ann follows close behind as we silently wander from room to room through the uneven light. The short crescent knives of her fingernails cut into my palm and wrist as I guide her through the maze of compact basement rooms. The hallways are narrow and dark, full of echoes.

"It's old," I say. "Probably one of the first houses built on the hill." I feel her hand stroking my arm, slowly, from shoulder to wrist. I don't turn to her, pretending not to notice, then she does it again. An ache rises up like a drug taking me, distracting the mind. I move on, leading her over the carpeted floors to the kitchen where she tugs my arm, turns me about, and comes at me with a moist and quivering mouth. Together we carefully and slowly collapse against the subterranean floor, then maniacally undress each other before the battered cabinets. She swings a short muscular leg over my hip, then carefully lowers herself, her weight descending purposefully.

"I like this house already," I say breathlessly. She doesn't say anything, but her mouth, I see, is smiling through the vast hair. Her eyes are rolled back in an effort of concentration. I am ripe for this and have been for a long time. As our bodies concuss I begin to feel the symptoms of my heart obstructing, an unambiguous dizziness rising up in my head. The palpitations gradually intensify, but I can't help myself. I don't care if I die like this. In fact, nothing could please me more. Dr. Epstein's voice comes to me full of foreboding, warning me against vigorous exercise, reminding me of the threat of sudden death. The voice is immediately dismissed as my vision grows clouded, the heart palpitates rabidly, and my body is consumed with that infinitely pleasant ache.

A few minutes later she lies against my chest, her warm moist skin cooling in the fractured light. I love the informality of lying naked together on a kitchen floor. Outside is the muted noise of a small city, inside is the buzz of flies between a shade and a dirty glass pane. As she lies on my chest, quiet and reflective, her shoulder curled into my ribs, I imagine she is assessing the damage done by reckless impulse. She should never have allowed herself this, a decision has been made: she has chosen to love *me*. I secretly turn this over in my mind.

"My heart began to palpitate a little," I murmur into the ceiling. "I got a little dizzy."

"That made you dizzy?" I feel her breath thrust against my skin.

"That did it."

"I felt a little dizzy too," she says, her voice lazy. "But it wasn't because of a weak heart."

Through the undergraduate years our lives enmesh, we become lovers. That fall she moves into the house, along with a retinue of friends I met in the dormitory and at SDS meetings. The household becomes a gathering hall for like-minded students—ardent revolutionaries, those who share a highly romanticized vision of the future and dismiss the present and past for all its inexplicable human folly.

Beneath the murky light of a paisley lampshade, a roommate, Carl, threads tiny glass beads together into a necklace, while another separates stems from plump and fragrant marijuana buds tangled into a bale. The air is stagnant with plumes of blue smoke spiraling out of ceramic incense trays, and a thick ragged joint passed between whitened forefingers and thumbs. Homeless men spend the night on the floor, bringing with them bags of Methedrine, which they inject into the thin blue veins of their forearms. At first it is novelty, a magnified view into the routine of junkies—leather tourniquets constricted about biceps, the geography of veins coming into relief as they run up the dirty forearm like lightning bolts. This masochistic affinity for needles I will never understand.

As their population grows, the times grow stranger. I feel no kinship, no empathy for these lost people. I am afraid of the drugs, afraid for my heart. I see the group experiment with poppers, the amyl nitrate the doctors at the NIH tried to burst my heart with as a teenager. I wag my head. They take much for granted, their health in particular, something I will never tolerate.

Then one morning in the spring of '70 I awake early. Ann is

curled into a compact question mark, her cheek and temple oc-
cupying the impression of the pillow I just left. The sun is low,
yellow and red bands of light come through new cottonwood foliage, imposing a strange color on the windowpane. I take in the
light while sitting on an edge of the bed, every now and then
glancing back to Ann as she sleeps, her mind lost in dreams,
then back toward the window. That static serenity where noise
ceases to be noise. Vague equilibrium.

Eventually I emerge from our bedroom. On the worn and
shiny Oriental rug are a half-dozen sleeping figures, some quivering in the morning chill, their minds twice removed in a drug
coma and sleep. Paraphernalia is scattered on the shallow coffee
table, abandoned as the party died in a rush during the small
hours of morning. The curtains are drawn, all sunlight
squelched. The pungent fumes of spent marijuana and hashish
seem to emanate from the obscure pattern of the rug. The musty
stench, the imprecise light of a Dutch opium den.

I pick a delicate path to the kitchen through the maze of unconscious bodies. Outside my Irish setter Gidget is curled
within the shade of her dog house, her chain tangled about her
body. From the kitchen window I can see her pale amber coat
twitching in sleep. In a corner of the kitchen beside the Art Deco
Frigidaire stands a tall bag of dog food. I take her bowl, dunk it
into the dark mouth of the bag, and scoop out a portion. When I
remove the bowl I see something strange. A syringe. A very dirty
syringe with the needle exposed. I lift it up to the light and see
traces of Methedrine solution pooled against the rubber plunger.
I set it down on the counter, take Gidget her food where she lies
in the shade, then watch her emerge from sleep to the happy
sight of a full dinner bowl. I watch her for a while, slowly losing
my temper over what I found inside. An image of Jessica sitting
on the lid of a toilet seat fills my mind, her dress pulled up to her
hip, the faint expression of dread as she exposes another needle. I

feel myself quietly losing control. The picture of selfish, self-satisfied pleasure cloaked beneath the shaggy beard of a junkie, their intolerance for order, their decision not to feel. I hate them. Their politics are a charade, they sense no calling.

When I return to the house, it's with a clamor. I beat a cookie pan against the walls, against sleeping heads. I shout that I want them all out now, that if they don't leave, I'm calling the cops. Their eyes loll in their skulls like the lazy eyes of livestock, sick, yellow, dull. When they slowly come to I lift them by the back of the collar and haul them out the front door where they collapse in a heap.

Eventually Carl appears, asking what the fuss is all about as he wipes sleep from his eyes.

"I found a Methedrine syringe in the dog food, Carl. I want these guys out of here now."

He massages his temples with his fingertips. In a weary voice he says, "Bob, they have no where to *go* . . . "

"That's not correct, Carl." I am yelling now. "They have no where to *stay*. They can't stay here. They can *go* wherever they like, anywhere at all. They just can't *stay* here."

And so that morning they leave, wandering about the town and campus until they find another house of college students looking for an accelerated means of procuring experience, cultivating it, growing it, like it were hair. Perhaps this morning is the end of my idealism, my belief that all people are inherently good, even junkies. Later I will come to believe that most people are capable of selfish ill-will at best, that the human heart is deeply and universally flawed. Not until I feel I have seen it all, not for some years to come, will I arrive at my final conclusion that anyone is capable of just about anything.

As lovers Ann and I sequester ourselves in our room where we lie together re-creating a small universe as lovers are inclined to do. I recall her lying on her belly with textbooks fanned out before a bright radius of lamplight. A pair of flannel boxer shorts and a V-neck T-shirt part at the small of her back, revealing the taut definition, the shallow crevice pouring into the nape of her buttocks. My hand blindly searches the sinuous shapes while she goes on aimlessly studying biology.

Through thick and thin we remain lovers. We come to share a past, a history we collect through the school years like a wonderful and terrifying booty shared out by simple and naive thieves. We see the world change, and witness each other change in it. But there is always the inability to make forecasts with conviction. After two years of life together, she moves to Denver, which lies forty-five minutes away, in order to attend nursing school. Yet we remain attached. Like all young and naive lovers, we are doomed in small ways from the very beginning. I learn something: anything that begins simply and innocently never stays that way for very long.

15

The sun is tenacious. A short bundle of one-page résumés in my hand collects perspiration and conforms to the shell-like shape of my palm. The concrete parking lot and pavement deflect sunlight and heat, cars lurch down the street, the cycle of combustion interrupted by vapor lock. A hot day in a big western city.

As the doors to the hospital part, the incoming stream of people is met with cool dry processed air. In the lobby I sit for a moment to recover, then go to a wall chart that maps the various departments. I write down the three-dimensional coordinates of cardiology, biochemistry, anatomy, surgery . . .

The first stop is Dr. Blount's office, as he is the chief of cardiology, and I know where his office is. He is my in, I tell myself. If all else fails, I have a sympathetic ear in Dr. Blount. I take the elevator up to the fourth floor, then head down the network of hallways where I meet him near another bank of elevators.

In one hand a short stack of papers is fanned out like playing cards, in the other are three metal clipboards. Around his neck the familiar Leatham stethoscope is casually strung. He is speaking quickly and loudly to another doctor down the hall, with the ease and confidence of a man in his own kitchen. When the conversation ends, he turns, our eyes meet, and his expression displays pleasant surprise.

He asks how I've been, how school is going. I tell him my heart is behaving no better or worse, really, and that I've graduated. I want to go to medical school and am looking for a job in some field of medical research in the meantime. I want to be a doctor. Can he help me, I ask, handing him my résumé.

"Sure, sure," he says, scanning my meager accomplishments.

"If you could just keep me in mind."

"I'll send this around, Bob."

The conversation returns to my heart as we head aimlessly down the hall. Through the course of college he has witnessed my rapid physical deterioration. I walk slowly now, resting often, and never run. Sports, even ease of movement, are part of a distant past. The conversation circuitously moves on to my plans, my obsession with cardiology, how it is the only professional interest I will ever have. He firmly pats my shoulder to acknowledge my conviction, then tells me to keep him abreast of my progress in the job hunt. But he must be off now. He pauses a moment and looks me over, inspecting my general health, while I read the keen solicitude in his eyes. Very warm and proper. A New England gentleman. I thank him and say I'll be by for a checkup next month, and I'm off to the next department.

All day long I go from door to door with my prefabricated address: Hi, my name is Bob Pensack. Last semester I graduated from the University of Colorado and am now looking to get into medical research here at the hospital. Would you care to . . . Hopelessness quickly descends upon the day. No one is interested, most can't even pretend to be. Toward evening I stop in at the department of surgery and ask for the chairman. The secretary immediately introduces me to Dr. Thomas Starzl, to whom I simultaneously give my perfunctory address and hand a résumé. I'm not quite prepared to speak, but I do so, awkwardly, a little rattled by his suffer-no-fools demeanor. He is slender and startlingly intense, his brown eyes absorbing the information, lifting it from the page. A busy man in a hurry. My delivery is skittish, my résumé outlandishly simple and common. My face flushes as he focuses on each item, the blood rising hot and carmine against my cheeks. I imagine his thoughts, the chief of surgery, as he reads the token phrases, *pre-med student, dean's list '68–'72, objective: admittance into an American medical school.* He must be laughing to himself. I silently beg, Please be a gentleman.

'Why don't I introduce you to Paul Taylor, our organ procurement officer," he says, his face down, a forefinger and thumb cradling the chin.

He walks off down the hallway and I follow in his wake, my skin chilled, fighting any display of surprise. He leads me to a small room where a black man in a white medical jacket is worrying over a stack of computer-processed data.

"Paul, I'd like you to meet Bob Pensack. Bob's interested in kidney and liver transplantation and wants to know about what's available in the animal research lab at the V.A."

I am beside myself. Dr. Starzl watches us exchange a tentative handshake, then pats my shoulder and leaves the room. A busy man in a hurry.

Two weeks later I receive a phone call from Paul Taylor early in the morning. Ann's body is sprawled across the sheets, her arm slung about my waist, when his serious voice pierces the static of sleep. Dr. Starzl has an opening in the kidney and liver transplant department if I'm still interested. I would dialyze patients waiting on kidney transplant lists, prepare dogs for liver and kidney transplantation, and assist in the production of an experimental drug, an immunosuppressant, called Anti-Lymphocyte Globulin (ALG). When could I start?

"Tonight," I tell him. I pretend to be serious. My heart is pounding now.

"Be here at 9:00 A.M. Wednesday." And he ends the conversation with a click.

16

A curious way to make a living. In the early morning the immunologist gives me a small metal case of pear-shaped vials of
human lymphocytes, white blood cells. In a Ford half-ton
pickup I drive over the undulations of prairie to a ranch just
beyond the edge of Broomfield, a small Colorado town. The purple silhouette of flatirons defines the horizon to the west, to the
east lies the perceptible curve of the earth as it capitulates to an
immense sky. In between are golden-brown wheat and hay
fields, a few scattered ranches and hamlets.

I arrive with the metal box beside me on the bench seat, along
with a collection of hypodermic needles. I meet the veterinarian
at the stable where he keeps a rather mangy palomino in a stall
with blinders over her eyes. We greet one another in the cool
darkness of the barn and quietly go about our business. The vet
is taciturn, unconvinced of the ethics in what we are doing, but
he has a job to do. He wears a small, bent and dirty Stetson over
his Indian-black hair. He is very much a part of the landscape,
especially in this barn, with its sharp smell of livestock. After
pulling the bridle over her limber ears, he tells me in a soft voice
that she's ready.

I open the metal lid and prepare the syringe in the poor light
and musty smells, and approach the horse. The head, the shape of
a milk bottle, sags from the neck. The vet wordlessly points out a
thick proud muscle standing out from the shoulder, and I part

the gray coat with my fingertips and jab the needle in at a blunt angle. The horse shimmies and gently brays as needle after needle of human lymphocytes are injected. Soon the job is done, and I drive for thirty minutes back to Denver.

That evening when I return home from work I find Ann's car parked on the street before my apartment. She is visiting, but neither as a girlfriend nor former girlfriend. Though we no longer live together, we haven't the will nor the ill-feelings toward one another necessary for a clean breakup. We are still lovers. We talk on the sofa that night after an informal dinner of left-over lasagna and salad. The job and Dr. Starzl dominate the conversation.

"The man is historical, Ann. He performed the first successful human liver transplant back in '67. He's one of the godfathers of transplant medicine."

"So what do you do for him."

"Today I injected an old mare with human white blood cells."

"Why?" She is appalled.

I attempt to explain the arcane science as she lies back deep into the sofa, a wineglass balanced between her fingers. She is serene but intensely interested. A ceiling fan twirls over the darkened room, stirring the air.

Transplant patients—people with grafts from nonrelated donors—require drugs that keep their body's immune system from attacking the donor organ. The body senses the otherness of its presence, that it is not of the body, just as it does a common virus. These drugs work by suppressing the immune system so that it is unable to attack the organ so vigorously. But it also lessens the body's ability to attack any common virus as well, so the treatment must be approached delicately.

It is a precarious balance. The chemistry is analogous to the politics of warfare: the enemy of my enemy is my brother. To produce the immunosuppressant, we inject a horse (because it is a large mammal) with human lymphocytes, which the *horse's* immune system recognizes as foreign. It responds by producing an antibody that attacks the human white blood cells as we continue to inject more of the lymphocytes through the course of several weeks. During that time the levels of these antibodies in the horse's circulatory system rise. Once a week I go out to the ranch with a sixty cc syringe and draw the horse's blood, then take the sample to the immunologist to measure the immune system's response to the human lymphocyte injection. Once the horse's body has produced enough antibodies against the white blood cells, I will bleed the horse to death, collecting its blood. The blood will be pumped into gigantic barrels which I will take to a lab in Denver where it is spun down in a centrifuge. The horse's antibodies are separated from the red and white blood cells, and collected in the form of a serum. The serum is eventually administered to transplant patients, and their own lymphocytes suppressed. The drug is called Anti-Lymphocyte Globulin (ALG).

"Ingenious," I say, smiling. "The enemy of my enemy is my brother."

Her jaw is relaxed, hanging open. She is at once appalled and amazed. She doesn't speak. Finally, she says, "So, what else do you do," as if afraid of the answer.

"I'm raising a chimp."

"Why would *you* be raising a chimp?"

"I don't know."

"You know." The remark is intended as an accusation.

Surgeons from all over the world converge upon our small department—Japanese, Israeli, Russian, German, French. There is an electric excitement not present anywhere else in the hospital, and Dr. Starzl is at the white-hot center. The man I had handed my simple résumé three weeks ago is not merely the chief of surgery at another academic hospital. He is perfecting the most complex procedures in transplant medicine, which are still in the pioneer stages. He has organized the protocol for organ procurement, and has had a hand in authoring the sensitive legislation concerning brain death.* These are just a few of his larger-than-life accomplishments. He is of course controversial on a grand scale.

One afternoon Paul Taylor enters the lab and approaches me ominously as I feed the chimp bananas. His expression is grim, he doesn't speak for a moment, as if trying to rattle me with the pause. Finally he speaks, but with reservation.

"They're wheeling a two-and-a-half-year-old girl into the OR for a liver transplant as we speak," he says. "If you're really interested in observing something like this, I'd suggest you get over to the OR right away."

"Of course," I say, amazed he would ask.

"Now, it won't be pretty," he warns. He approaches me, his brow stern, severe, as I stand next to the cage, a peeled banana in my hand. He gazes into my eyes without speaking to convey the seriousness of what I will witness. "You'll be standing for sixteen to twenty hours. A little girl's life will be on the line in there, so *stay out of the way.*"

I head directly to the OR, take a fresh pair of surgical greens out of the closet, then go to the men's locker room where a small clique of foreign surgeons speaks in fragmented English. As I dress beyond a partition of metal lockers, I quietly listen as they

---

*When someone is brain dead he or she has suffered a complete and irreversible loss of brain stem reflexes. These are the reflexes that control functions like blood pressure, respiration, and other vital activities of the body. For donation to occur, artificial life support systems are used to maintain heartbeat and breathing since the brain can no longer do so. If these support systems are removed, all vital body functions stop. Brain death is irreversible, and is an acceptable medical, ethical and legal principle.

plot a strategy for what they are about to do. They speak a technical jargon in a language that isn't native to any of them. Soon they file out, heads bowed in thought. Once dressed, I enter the OR suite where they have assembled around the young recipient's body where it lies beneath a broad sphere of surgical light. The crest of her abdomen is bathed in a golden disinfectant, a tiny endotracheal breathing tube has been inserted into her windpipe. In the suite across the hall lies the donor baby, brain dead, its small abdomen parted, the precious organs glistening beneath Starzl's magnified gaze. The room has taken on the bizarre air of solemnity and deadly seriousness. I walk from one room to the other, trying to pick up on exactly what is taking place, how the surgeries are orchestrated. I am nervous, the adrenaline running clean and potent. I just want to stay out of the way, yet at the same time I am vitally interested. I am not a tourist here, though I can't help but consider the setting a kind of metaphor for war, a war at which I have a box seat. Somehow this has something to do with my being; I feel this viscerally. The sense has metaphysical force.

As I stand upon a short stool next to the anesthesiologist's station where the donor baby lies, an OR nurse wanders toward me and stands at my side.

"They're nearly finished harvesting the liver," she says, her eyes on the small bloody scene that lies beneath the surgeons' fingers.

"Harvesting?"

"Removing the organs."

"Ahh. That's a peculiar term."

"I thought so once. But through the years I've concluded that it's very appropriate." Her eyes are moist above the blue surgical mask.

Two surgeons work quickly and quietly on either side of the short table, their heads almost touching. Once the organ is separated from the donor, the dark crimson mass is carefully placed in a stainless steel pan where it soaks in nutrients, then it is brought at once to the suite across the hall where the recipient lies, anesthetized, her abdomen gaping upon a table. The two surgeries have been carefully choreographed so that the act of harvesting dovetails into the act of replacement. The surgery is intricate. Dozens of tiny blood vessels must be sewn together between the donor organ and the recipient. Gradually it becomes hers. Through the grueling hours of the night I carefully observe Starzl at work, and come to understand that I am not witnessing an ordinary man. It seems he was born for this task, that he was genetically engineered to solve this vast mystery himself. The divine intervention is even present in his physical makeup; his fingers are long and thin, almost feminine, spiderlike, instruments ideally suited for the tedious and intricate job of weaving together tiny blood vessels, reconnecting human beings, making them whole.

Through the night, the following morning, and well into the afternoon, I observe the bitter progress from where I stand upon the short stool. I become dizzy with sleeplessness, the room quivers under me as I walk, yet the surgeons implacably work on. Every couple of hours a surgeon will come in to relieve Starzl. After a few explanatory words, he brusquely heads through the OR doors to the lounge where he sits himself on the modern vinyl upholstery of a sofa, stares into the brightness of a single rectangular window, then carefully lights and smokes cigarette after cigarette. His eyes wander across the tar-and-gravel rooftop of the hospital, then onto the turning foliage of residential Denver. After three or four smokes, his slender neck arches back against the cushion, and he is lost in sleep for ten or fifteen minutes. Then his eyes will suddenly open and he is wide-awake, looking fresh and aggravated, ready for another long pull at the operating table.

By 4:00 P.M. the following day they are wheeling the girl on a gurney into the elevator, which will deliver her to the ICU. Eventually she will arrive at the clinical research ward to recover among the growing population of other kidney and liver transplant recipients.

After the surgery I drive home to Boulder for an uninterrupted twelve-hour sleep. The phone rings in my dreams, then ceases. When I finally awake at dawn the following morning, I put on a large pot of coffee, shower, then call Ann to tell her what I've seen.

"It's your man with the chimp."

"Where have you been?" Her voice is small, sleepy.

"I watched an eighteen-hour liver transplant. A little girl, two and a half years old."

"I called and called . . ." I hear her head collapse against the pillow. "You're going home soon, aren't you?"

"For Thanksgiving. Not for another week."

I proceed to explain the process, though she's too tired to be interested, then let her go back to sleep. After a casual morning of reading the paper, watching the news and fortifying my blood with hot black Colombian coffee, I drive back to the hospital and go directly to the clinical research ward only to find the girl is still in the ICU. Even under the best of circumstances, she won't arrive here for forty-eight hours, a nurse tells me.

But three days later I hear she has made it. Several times a week I go there to dialyze kidney patients, a process that takes four or five hours. During my breaks I walk to her room where she lies beneath bright lights among a throng of stuffed animals, doctors, nurses and family. Her prognosis, I discover, is excellent. She has years ahead of her.

•   •   •

I come to know most of the patients I dialyze, as the process is slow and generally relaxed, allowing time for drawn-out conversation. Most have had their brush with death, a topic I am naturally drawn to. The macabre is touched with small wishes and modest considerations of hope. But there is one patient I don't come to know, though his image will continue to haunt me as his kidney slowly betrays him, poisoning then eventually infecting his blood. His name is Steve, the only black patient on the ward, and he wants to go to medical school. Through the course of a month he gradually loses his grip on consciousness and is continually on the verge of slipping into a coma. The heavy doses of immunosuppressants that are required to rescue his newly transplanted kidney from rejection has left him wide-open to devastating infection. His body is septic, he grows frail, his eyes sunken within the dark skin. One day I knock on the door to his room and enter, only to find his bed perfectly made, his pillow fluffed. I ask the nursing staff about him, but no one knows what happened since they weren't on duty when he left. The easiest conclusion to come to is that he died, being not at all uncommon on this ward. This is where the heady work of miracles is broken by the shadow left by the dying. What I need is a vacation.

17

There are the familiar ripe hues of early fall, east coast colors. The air is dry and cool, crêpe paper streamers from Friday's homecoming game bleed into the moist turf of the Newark Academy football field. John Ritota, his younger brother, Ted, John Kimmel, Bill Guenther, along with old friends of Newark Academy and myself are walking over the shallow crown of the field, deciphering what has changed, what has stayed the same through the course of four years. Together we collect the remains of our shared past. Reunions become modest attempts at reconstructing and preserving a skeleton of days.

Under my arm I carry a leather football, which the chilly air has made hard. We divide ourselves into two teams, then a coin is flipped for the kickoff. I balance the ball beneath my purpled right forefinger, John Ritota nods, and the metallic hardness leaves in a rush, suspended in the cold gray sky. The bright colors of rugby shirts labor over the field, cheeks redden against the cold. Through the afternoon we play hard, exaggerating our new physical limitations, our mature deficiencies. We remark how each has gained weight, point out breathlessness as though it were a badge of honor. The unspoken suggestion is that my own physical deterioration is a natural condition of aging, that I am just one of the boys. I find comfort in this solidarity, this collective denial. Cold air stings the bridge of my nose and penetrates deep into the forehead. The heart surges, then retreats as I alternately sprint then bow down, sinking my head between my knees. The mind clears once flooded with fresh blood, and I'm off again, trying to keep pace with the game. Just one of the boys.

Smoking chimneys fill the residential skyline as the day grows late. The sun lowers, dull and very orange, seemingly distant and cool, but the game goes on, energized by the strange light. The ball is hiked into my parted hands, and John Ritota goes deep, fantastically deep. I mimic a play-action, curl out toward the chalk sidelines upon the grass as I am pursued by John Kimmel, and arc the ball through the orange sky. The ball leaves my scope of vision as I focus on the whir of John's long legs, the mad flapping of his red and blue rugby shirt like a flag in the wind. The ball drifts over his right shoulder and is tugged against his chest. I throw my hands up in disbelief then charge down the field with my head in my hands, skipping and jumping, the empty bleachers rushing by my corner vision, the steady succession of faded chalk lines, the rising moon suspended in the dull light. I carry the mad flutter in my chest as I run downfield. Then sudden darkness. A strange and terrible dream. My arms jerk wildly in tonic and clonic seizures as I lose consciousness and my friends watch on, helplessly, in horror.

Then light. My eyelids bat like butterfly wings, I am jostled, my heart pounds out of sync. Deep in the seat of my jeans I feel a cold wetness.

Bobby . . . Bobby . . .

I see the faces of friends against the darkening sky above me, I smell the earthy smell of turf and sweat. I tell myself I am alive, blink my eyes, then say aloud, I pissed in my pants.

Bobby . . . Bobby . . .

Again, I tell myself I am alive.

• • •

Through the glass pane I can hear the dry leaves scraping against the concrete as they are blown down the street. The glass rattles when the wind picks up. The day is cold and gray, the threat of rain constant as a seamless sheet of low clouds rolls in from the coast. I hear the phone ringing downstairs, and a few minutes later Dad quietly enters the guest bedroom to tell me Richard is on the line.

"I hear you wet your pants."

"Gillette called it atrial fibrillation."

"You'll be okay. I know it's scary, but it's only the upper chambers."

"Gillette said it was compatible with life. I like that. They just sent me home to bed," I say. "My heart didn't feel normal until this morning, like it was out of sync."

"You'll be okay, Bob. Hang in there"

"It's getting worse, anyway. Gillette made an appointment for me at the NIH for next month."

"Still, it's the upper chambers. I've had it lots of times. It scares the shit out of you, but you won't die."

This is the brother I love, the voice of a sympathetic Greek oracle, my prophet. Our bond is deepened at such times. However, his moods can be pendulous, and he will often dismiss the subject of our shared illness as though he simply wants to pretend we are free of it. But not now.

Three days later Dad drives me to the airport. He tries to be reassuring by guiding the conversation around my heart to other subjects such as my job, my chances of getting into medical school. What happened to me on the football field was a quirk, I just need to be more careful. Again, it is dismissed as being compatible with life.

Back in Boulder I carry the memory of the event about with me like a secret, a genetic humiliation. For the first time I make the conscious connection that I have the same disease as my mother, and that I will die soon. I am twenty-three years old and dying. At unexpected moments I have powerful and vivid recollections of looking into the empty gray sky as I lay on the field, mentally praying, please god, please god, please please please don't let me die like my mother.

After my return, work takes on a grave seriousness. I need to get into medical school, I feel as though my life will eventually depend upon it as the disease progresses. Besides, no other work interests me.

Then one night late in the fall, just a few days before my trip to the NIH, I receive a call at 1:00 A.M. from Paul Taylor.

"You need to get to the animal lab and prepare the chimp for anesthesia."

"What's going on?" I ask, not fully awake.

"Starzl's transplanting his liver into a man tonight. He can't find a human donor, and the guy has only a few hours left."

I glance at the clock, looking for something that will firmly ground this conversation in either dreams or reality.

"Get here as soon as you can," he says sternly. The phone clicks.

A vigorous excitement accompanies me on the drive to Denver, the excitement of an Apollo moonshot. This is one of the first cross-species transplants ever attempted, this is history. The chimp, I have heard, was once the property of NASA. Starzl procured him from a military base in San Antonio a few years ago, where it is rumored it was an astronaut. At any rate, his liver is about to become human in a few hours since a donor can't be found.

The chimp is asleep in his cage when I arrive. I speak softly to him as I approach, telling him what he's doing in the name of Science. Once he stirs, he is instantly alert, swinging about the bars by his long thin hairy arms.

I administer a tranquilizer with a hypodermic needle, then

shave and prep his abdomen, and soon he is being hauled on a child's gurney down to the OR, his eyes sleepy and puzzled. The doctors there take him into the OR suite, and I never see him again. I harbor no remorse. He may give a man the gift of a few years, I tell myself.

A few days after the surgery I fly out of Denver for the NIH in Bethesda. There they want to do a complete study of my heart, another right and left heart cath, along with a slew of noninvasive procedures. After four days of lurking about the chambers, Dr. Epstein presents me with a choice. Either they can dramatically increase my prescription of Inderal, or I could opt for an experimental surgery that would thin the muscular septum of my heart, allowing it to fill and empty more completely when exercising. What I have, he explains, is a muscle-bound heart.

The news stuns my senses. I will die as my mother died. Now I am sure. Though it is left unsaid, the surgery will eventually become necessary, as I am already taking immense doses of Inderal. This much I can figure out for myself. I leave the NIH with several large bottles of the drug in my suitcase, and the certainty that this temporary measure isn't going to prove much. The surgery is imminent. Ann and I now lead utterly separate lives since she has returned to Oregon, and there is no one to share this news with. No one at all.

When I return to Denver late in the week, I visit the clinical research ward and ask about the man with the chimp's liver. He died, a nurse tells me, from acute rejection. His xenophobic body didn't take to the foreign genetic structure of the liver. She appears sad and hurt, her trust in medical science shattered.

"It was a long shot," I say. "Maybe someday."

She rolls her eyes. "It just seemed a little . . . I don't know . . . crazy."

The story will never reach the press, and the world will go about with its business. And meanwhile I've got my own to tend to. That evening after work I walk out to my mailbox. Inside I see there is a large envelope from the University of Colorado Medical School. My heart quickens, the familiar dizziness washes through me. I walk to a wooden public bench and open the envelope within the blue light of an electric streetlamp. Inside are several forms, and a letter congratulating me on my acceptance into their medical school. Immediately I feel tears rising toward my eyes, my heart palpitating. After two years I am finally going to be a doctor, I say to myself. Then aloud: "I am going to be a doctor." I stand up, firmly gripping the package in both hands as a cold wind sweeps through the streets. I walk back to the house beneath the glow of streetlamps, and the howl of the wind against the city. "Finally," I say. In the night air there is the faint pang of irony.

Three days later I receive a letter from San Francisco.

Dear Bob,

I also want to add my personal sincere congratulations and best wishes to you for your success in breaking through the medical school monopoly.

I hope that you will always keep in mind the importance of working to break down all monopolies and achieving the goal of equal rights for *all* and special privileges for *none*.

Love,
Richard

FLESH WOUNDS

18

The light is sourceless, the auditorium simply glows. This aspect alone casts it as modern. There is the electric hum of nervous conversation, talk for the sake of talk. When the dean enters the small door beneath the vast periodical chart, the room rustles vigorously, then quiets. Once he addresses the podium and taps the microphone with a forefinger, the room is silent, producing the aural sensation of being underwater.

He begins with congratulations, a welcome, then confident reassurance that all of us, all one hundred ten, will be doctors in four years. The process of natural selection has already occurred. Do not concern ourselves with fear of failure; the school has already invested considerable money in each of us. Today, in the fall of 1974, we are about to embark on the richest intellectual experience known to mankind, we will hold a special place in society—as healers. We are granted permission from this point forward to begin feeling significant.

But failure is the only thing on anyone's mind. The closed society we form is driven by fear of it. It is an absurd but basic motive. With the assurances we received the first day, one might expect a more casual atmosphere. But the compulsive personalities that delivered everyone here cannot be turned on and off like a light switch. Compulsion is bred-in-the-bone.

I doubt many in this anxious coterie are driven only by an altrustic need to heal, to remove another's pain, create a new landscape for living. Not that I am certain it matters. The practice of medicine is a craft as well as an art in that it requires skill at the bidding of intuition. It is the ability to intuit invisible and complex scenes that comes after thousands of hours of obsessive labor. Intuition is the child of the overprepared mind, and we are all determined to acquire this elusive sense.

In my case I can't help but think I am unique: I have grandiose dreams of curing my secret illness, and the only way to do that is to become an M.D. first. Though the dream is a romantic one, it is inextricably woven in with my own elemental fear of failure. I promise to become my own model doctor, my own best patient. I will learn to save myself, I will endure the greatest trauma to do it. But first I must become a doctor. Failure and death are an intricate tangle of thorns in the loom of my imagination. Academic failure amounts to a premature death.

Nevertheless, the sheer volume of work expected is startling. What I did in college through the gentle course of a semester is done in a single week. If you do not cram each night, you quickly become hopelessly behind. But the sudden influx of information produces hope, a new trust in the ability of medical science to heal the human body. The language of medicine becomes a kind of Sanskrit, a self-referring vocabulary that quickly separates us from the rest of the world, the world beyond medicine. We eat together, drink, smoke, stay awake and sleep together. Our skin fades to a pale shade of yellow through the seasons. The intimacy is incestuous, but satisfying by virtue of its intensity. Friends from college quickly become part of a messy and incomplete past simply because the singular focus of this strange new curriculum demands it. As our scope of human experience is narrowed, lives merge into each other, our successes and failures become mutual.

With the advent of the second semester comes anatomy class, an academic forum that represents the very essence of medicine, with all its casual disregard of taboos and everyday squeamishness. We are divided into groups of four, each of which is presented with a human cadaver. As we dissect the preserved flesh and bone through the blur of days and nights, we share the camaraderie of battle-tested soldiers, with all their weary pride and arrogance.

The study is laden with jokes, an emotional response to cloak the anxiety of touching and cutting preserved human flesh. At first there is conjecture of the life of the cadaver, the history she lived, and death, which quickly decays into morbid humor. She becomes an elaborate and haunting fictional character. It becomes unclear to me after being awake through the small hours of the morning who the ghosts are, who are the cadavers, who are the living dead. Despite wearing gloves during the dissections, there is never any ridding the skin of the stench of formaldehyde. It is there when we date each other, go to bars together, sleep together, always the image of an exquisite cadaver.

It is during these years that my fascination for the anatomy of the human heart becomes a full-blown obsession. I carry a secret concealed in my chest that I share with no one in spite of the environment of intimacy. Apart from microbiology, neuroanatomy, physiology, biochemistry, I dwell on its structure and nature. I become a cardiologist long before becoming a doctor, studying all the primitive literature available on IHSS, reading the basics of cardiology. The science becomes a kind of absolution offering the promise of correction.

I take an elective class called "Auscultation of the Heart," a course in which we learn the heart sounds by listening to phonograph recordings of normal and pathological organs. Within a few weeks I master the science by listening to the pathological sounds of my own when feeling weak or light-headed. The motivation to learn has a new physical source, a precise and distinct sound, not merely a mental compulsion as with other students.

But through that first year of medical school, the symptoms

worsen. Nightmares haunt my sleep, driving the mind, wakeful and alert, deep into the night. I grow anxious around the clock, insomnia bleeds the day of its usual energy. Sometimes during mild exercise, even during an exam or after a large meal, the symptoms intensify, producing an audible murmur when examined with a stethoscope. During the worst of these times I have hurried to Dr. Blount's office across the street in a panic, my eyes tearing, voice breaking, certain my life is about to come to an abrupt and lonely end. When I arrive I try to appear casual, though I'm scared, my heart pounding madly. He sits me down on an office chair, lifts my shirt, then listens in the broad silence. I observe the concern etched in the lines traversing his forehead as he captures the strange noise in his large ears. Finally he lifts his head and says, "Now that's an impressive murmur, Bob."

"Whenever I eat a steak, or any large meal it happens."

He laughs gently.

"I'm not sure that would be enough to produce a murmur like that." His brow is skeptical.

"It has to have something to do with it. Happens all the time."

"I'm just not convinced that alone could do . . . *that*," he says, pointing with a certain alarm at my heart. He can offer little more than reassuring words before sending me on my way back to the lab.

After a series of such visits, we devise a test to see whether or not it is the laborious digestion of food that is causing the murmur. Dr. Blount maintains his skepticism, while I am certain. Before I head home to eat, Dr. Blount listens to my heart, impressing in his memory the sound of a vague murmur, a sick heart at rest. Then I go home, light the fire beneath the metal stove grate, place a marinated slab of a New York steak into the dull black skillet, and listen to the sound of flesh against hot iron. The slab of meat fades from a crimson to burnished brown, and I take it from the skillet to my plate, then surround it with a cold leafy salad mixed with wedges of cucumber and tomato. I sit with my plate, steak knife and fork at the small wooden kitchen table and begin severing the tender meat. The marbled thickness dissolves in my mouth, flooding the senses with the primitive rapture of satisfying hunger. Midway through the meal I open the window at the far end of the apartment to allow in the calamity of the city, and usher out the rich blue smoke over the stove. The falsetto of Marvin Gaye floats from a neighbor's stereo, blotting out much of the noise.

After I've finished, I feel the implacable return of the symptoms, the dizziness that accompanies simple motion, the sense of a sick heart struggling to digest its body's fuel. I slowly make my way out of the apartment and head back to Dr. Blount's office deep within the hospital where he is waiting, the chrome tongs of his Leatham pinching into his lean neck.

Again, I sit down, he listens, and eventually shakes his head as he pulls the instrument from his ears and drapes it over his shoulders slumped in resignation.

"You're goddamn right, Bob. That's one impressive murmur." He doesn't look me in the eye, as he now has a new understanding of the extent of my heart's weakness.

The amount of blood that pools in my gut to digest a large meal takes away from the normal volume of blood returning to my heart with each beat. The less blood in my heart, the worse the obstruction becomes, blocking the flow on its mission to nourish the body with oxygen and nutrients. It is the obstruction that causes the audible sound, known as a murmur. Blount knows what this means, and it shows in his eyes: the thickened heart is now threatening my everyday existence.

In the face of the bad news, I feel supremely triumphant. That I can explain why I feel worse after a large meal is soothing. It validates the academic work I've done, validates my own worth as a future physician. The discovery is evidence that I can master this disease, come to know it so intimately that I will be able to survive with it. I am a spy in the house of my heart.

The following summer I take a research job in cardiology under the auspice of Dr. Steele, the chief of cardiology at the V.A. Hospital just down the street from the medical school. It is a good research job in that Dr. Steele's interests lie in innovation, serious academic work. Years ago he was instrumental in developing the first noninvasive technique for imaging the heart, using a nuclear isotope. This is cutting-edge cardiology; yet my job is simple. I inject these patients on the coronary care unit who have new infarcts (dead muscle as a result of a recent heart attack) with the isotope. The isotope is naturally absorbed by the newly dead muscle, enabling us to take a picture of the infarcted area, which is then enhanced by a computer. The new technology is significant, as it accurately depicts the area destroyed by the heart attack.

During the short hot summer I also spend much of my day in the heart cath lab, assisting in the very procedures I endured as a child and an adult. I feel a release, a false sense of confidence, like that of a graduate; I am no longer the patient, but fast on my way to becoming the doctor. I silently repeat to myself like a mantra that I shall remain the doctor. The confusion in my imagination is deeply reassuring, though it is based on a lie I unwittingly tell myself.

Once each week I also scrub in for open-heart surgery and witness the gaping carmine wound where the heart lies quivering and stunned in the parted cradle of ribs. I do not observe this scene and ask myself if this is to be me soon. I do not ask if I am witnessing my future. I have a different disease than these patients, a genetic illness that has nothing to do with plaque-laden coronary arteries, typical heart attacks. Nor can it be remedied with basic bypass surgery. Perhaps this is another deliberate confusion on my part, as I am completely capable of suppressing all awareness of identification I have with them. Again, I am the "doctor." Two different diseases, two different approaches to management.

Through the months, however, I begin to feel intense, pervasive feelings of nervousness, deteriorating concentration and memory. My nights are haunted with dreams that are metaphors for death. These symptoms always correspond with the deteriorating symptoms of my heart. As the symptoms worsen, the disease becomes impossible to conceal, and therefore necessary to talk about. Friends want to know, they want answers. And at times I want someone to share the pain with, but not a cardiologist, not my father, not even Richard. Ironically, the severity of my symptoms has surpassed his in many ways, my heart has grown even more muscle-bound. In a sense, I am now the oracle. And what could I tell friends that would calm me, make me feel I am not in this alone? I am in this alone. All alone.

19

She stands with her back to me in this lingering memory, the plump blond ponytail bobbing as she moves down a sunlit corridor, the lateral rays penetrating and refracting through her hair. She is the focus of all light. In her arms she carries a stack of medical textbooks against her sweater as if they needed protecting.

At age twenty-four Allison has forty-year-old surgeons mindlessly following her skirt through the hallways of the medical school. She receives phone calls, it is widely known, through the night from residents working across the street at the University Hospital. She likes dirty jokes, has a brilliant intellect, dresses like an uptown hooker and talks like one, too. She is also everything I am not: Protestant, blonde, blue-eyed, in the top five of her class at Harvard, and very close to her family who lives in New York.

In the beginning a certain distance is kept, mainly because I know she would have little incentive to become interested in someone like me. Of course I would like to think this distance is prompted by my own forbidding pride, but of course my pride has little to do with it.

Then one winter night at a party we exchange bawdy jokes over a bottle of scotch, something for which I discover she has a real passion, and come to know each other. Not long after that first night a love affair develops, a Roman candle love affair in that it is intense, colorful, and brief. What keeps us together is what brought us together in the first place—our humor, which is of the same irreverent vein. What will eventually tear us apart is so unusual it cannot be forecast. But it's this brief and brilliant interlude that is significant.

As the summer of '75 wears on, my heart disease steadily worsens. Yet, still few know of the secret I carry about with me in my chest, not even Allison. Then one day in class, a class we happen to share, I nervously raise my hand to ask the professor a question, and abruptly feel my heart obstructing. My forehead spins, my stomach rushes up my throat in a wave of nausea, just as it had on the football field two years ago. I manage to fire off the question before my head collapses in my hands parted on the wooden desk top. Then I hear my question being answered as though from a great distance while I lie still, and my heart struggles to relax. After class Allison is concerned and asks if I feel all right.

"I'm fine, really," I say, dismissing any more questions with a wave of the hand.

"You didn't seem fine five minutes ago."

"It's just a little queasiness. Nothing, really."

That afternoon I head across the street to Dr. Blount's office in the hospital to explain to him what happened.

"Performance anxiety," he says. His eyes are strangely grave.

"I get nervous, my system is flooded with adrenaline, and the heart obstructs," I say, as if reciting a poem.

"Exactly."

"The Inderal isn't working anymore."

"That's right."

"It's time for the surgery."

There's a long tortuous pause.

"Bob, it's time."

Ironically, I feel another wave of dizziness with the utterance

of those words. To this day they haunt me—*Bob, it's time . . .* Dr.
Blount places a hand on the crown of my bowed head and says, "I
don't know what else there is to do."

I know of the danger inherent in this experimental surgery.
It's called a septal myotomy and myectomy, which means my
heart will be stopped, a section of the septum pared away, allowing the chambers to fill and empty more completely. I also know
the surgery carries a one-in-five mortality rate. Blount knows
this as well. These are mathematics I cannot escape. There is of
course the possibility that they could accidentally damage the
part of the septum that governs the heart's pacing system, so I
may require a permanent electronic pacemaker. But there's only
an outside chance of that.

That night I invite Allison over to my apartment for dinner.
She arrives early with a small bottle of Chardonnay, and immediately assaults me with a volley of questions ranging from the personal to the clinical to the accusatory: Is it some sort of
cardiomyopathy? Were you ashamed to tell me? Is this the disease your mother died of? She displays the cocky confidence of
having pieced together a vast and intricate mystery. The staccato
of her speech immediately overwhelms, so I turn my back on her
voice and begin peeling away the lead seal from the cork on the
wine bottle. I involve myself in the task of sinking the chrome
corkscrew just off-center, spiraling it into the soft fleshy wood,
then carefully pry it from the throat of the bottle. Meanwhile her
talk gradually dies down. Once I've poured two glasses, there's a
momentary silence.

"I'm going to have open-heart surgery next month. A septal
myotomy and myectomy."

She stares across the kitchen, her blue eyes boring into mine.
The eyebrows pinch together, the tan neck extends.

More silence.

"I'll be leaving town for about six weeks or so," I say, looking away. I then lift both wineglasses by the stems, and, avoiding her stare, I approach her, offering the glass. "So, let's propose a toast. To rose-lipped maidens and lightfooted lads . . ."

She slowly floats toward me, then carefully smothers me in her hair and warmth. Her arms drift about my body, careful of the wine, but some does spill.

"Carefully, now. My cup runneth over," I say.

"Young man," she says slowly, but with a trace of agony in her voice, "your cup is cracked."

The next day I head to the dean's office before class to tell him I'll be away for a month or two, but that I plan to be back as soon as I'm able. The dean is shocked and concerned; he reassures me he'll make the transition as easy as possible for me, then asks about my disease, of which I tell him as he listens behind his broad oak desk with his chin resting contemplatively on the heel of his palm. I conclude the story with my need to announce the departure to not only the faculty, but also my class, and he warmly agrees.

So that afternoon, amid the glowing sourceless light of the auditorium where I was assured of becoming a doctor a year and a half ago, I wearily mount the dais and announce into the live microphone that I'll be leaving soon, and explain why. Then I leave the podium, and the lecture begins with a stunned silence.

The following week, the night before my departure for the NIH, I walk back from the library to my apartment. The night sky is dense with stars, the city eerily quiet. There is a harrowing clarity about the evening, as the darkness is broken by tiny incandescent lights. I stop on the sidewalk and look up into a black patch of sky to allow the stars to form any pattern they will against the darkness. My mind calms as they stare back, never organizing themselves into shapes or mythical characters—no Orion, no Andromeda, no Leo. Just a random glitter of lights against the darkness. After a few minutes I continue on, trying not to think, shutting out all pictures of bloody carnage I've witnessed on the surgical table, all images of bright and sterile landscapes. I fix my thoughts on the odor of woodsmoke present in the air as I cut through a lawn, my shoes sinking into sodden leaves and soil. I imagine scenes from sleepaway camp: the childhood terror of the hardwood forest at night that surrounded the camp, the smell of campfires, the wild flames, the warmth and security of community.

As I approach my apartment, my mind is miles and years away. The chill has leaked through my jacket and settled in my bones. I head through the entryway, sink the key into the lock and open it to the brilliant flash of the lights and the howl of voices. The stereo suddenly comes to life and my back is slapped, my shoulders hugged, then I'm led to the balcony where a plastic cup of scotch is thrust into my palm.

Within minutes I've shaken my gloom, and feel the jokes rising up in me like a hill. What I had contemplated with terrifying clarity just a few minutes ago, what I came to understand, how I came to see what I'm up against, the very mathematics of mortality, are now all distant thoughts. I sip on a scotch, then another and another. Eventually Allison appears from out of the crowd and swaddles me in her arms, spilling scotch onto her shoe.

"My cup runneth over again," I say over the clatter of music and voices.

"Your cup is cracked, Bobby."

The following morning she drives me to the airport where she happily carries my luggage to the ticket counter, and we say a long goodbye. Then I'm carried away, once again, watching the violet granite of the Rockies diminish within a glass oval as I soar eastward.

•   •   •

At the NIH I am placed on the cardiology ward where I meet other people roughly my own age who also have IHSS. During the long sunny days prior to the surgery I make my way down the narrow hallway to the solarium where we regularly exchange stories. There is no need for shame or fear, only the quiet satisfaction of camaraderie, the brand-new sense of recognizing yourself in others. The only other person I've ever met with IHSS is Richard, which has until now cast the disease as being extraordinarily rare and therefore deadly. The interest the NIH has held in IHSS has never failed to amaze me. Perhaps that is why I have had this wellspring of gratitude for this place; I am secretly moved by what I've understood to be philosophical and medical altruism on the part of the individuals who make up such institutions, filled with the certainty that these halls were built and staffed to relieve the suffering of Richard and Robert Pensack. But with this visit, I understand the atmosphere of individual caring is something of an illusion, and the result is of course a happy one. This disease, I now learn as I sit in a semicircle of patients, all connected to IV poles, is far less rare than I initially thought.

The stories we share are war stories, horrible little vignettes that have killed and maimed, leaving the survivors shaking with the fallen wonder of life's purpose. It slowly occurs to me that the tales are no different than those I've heard from acquaintances and friends of acquaintances who have returned from Vietnam. Both possess the same electric drama that terrifies, both raise the same elemental questions that pit the naked human will against oblivion. Yet the sharing of stories is soothing; there is no cause to pretend, to feel I am not normal, because here I am normal. There is also the security of being surrounded by doctors who have cared for me for nine years now—the best doctors on the planet. Considering the circumstances, I couldn't feel more safe.

Not long after the stories have begun, a short rotund man

with the jovial demeanor of Santa Claus approaches our small group in the solarium. He addresses me as though I should know him. Obviously he's a doctor, as he has a stethoscope strung about his neck, either a cardiologist or a surgeon. After a salvo of jokes and anecdotes, he introduces himself as Dr. Morrow, the surgeon who will perform my operation. He then heads to the corner of the room, selects a chair, which he drags in his wake, and joins our small party.

"So I see you've all had a chance to get acquainted," he says, smiling with a kind of abandonment that immediately puts me at ease.

"I thought I was the only person with this disease till yesterday," I say.

"That's pretty mutual all the way around," another patient announces, a southerner, indicating our semicircle with a lazy swirl of his finger.

Dr. Morrow's eyes retreat to his fingertips which he holds woven together in his lap. His mood seems to have suddenly turned meditative.

"That's the peculiar nature of IHSS," he says to no one in particular. I see beneath his lowered brow that he's still smiling.

After a long but calming pause, he addresses me specifically and explains what they have in mind for my surgery. Always, I notice, he speaks compassionately of what they *have in mind.*

"I understand you're fast on your way to becoming a physician?"

"I *was* fast on my way." I manage a smile.

"Ahh. Well, hopefully you'll soon be back in the classroom feeling better than ever. What we have in mind, as I'm sure you're aware, is a septal myotomy and myectomy. Of course you know the Greek for this: *my* being of the heart muscle, *otomy* being to cut into, *ectomy* to cut out. So we'll be removing a thin section of the septum."

"Right," I say looking over at the group who all hold lost expressions.

"Understand, we're not going to cure you," he begins, trying not to sound didactic. "We aren't going to take IHSS from your heart. Nor will we eliminate all the symptoms. We can, however, put an end to these dizzy spells." He raises a finger and says gently but emphatically: "Hopefully."

As the date of the surgery nears, I notice my behavior growing more erratic, my moods swinging more pendulously from the hopeful to the shadowy realm of gloom. I spend most of the long cold sunny days on my back in a private room with EKG wires taped in a broad tapestry about my chest, reading, eating, doing little other than trying to forget the knife and table that await me. Sometimes at night I see the narrow table beneath the large milky circle of light of a surgical lamp; beyond the perimeter of light is only darkness, a world of shadows. During the daylight hours I muse over what would be happening at school at that very moment, where each of my friends would be, what my lab partners are doing. I wonder which of the residents is following Allison's ponytail through the corridors.

Then the day before the surgery while pretending to read, my mind continues to roam across the continent. What happens next is an understandable phenomenon, particularly among those about to face what lies before me. Masturbation is the sterile child of anxiety, the joke we play on god. That afternoon as I spend but a few minutes lost in images of girlfriends, mental lovers, I feel my heart beginning to obstruct. I cannot see the ceiling for the images that fill the mind; the sensual obscures the everyday, the soft parade obscures the terror. Then suddenly there is the world with all its blunt surfaces. The door swings open, followed by the shuffling of shoes over the tile, and the voice of my nurse.

"Are you all right, Bob?"

My mind aches, my eyelids flutter as they struggle for control.

"Fine, fine," I say, curling my knees to my chest.

"The monitor showed your heart rate increasing." Her eyes are wide with wonder and surprise.

"It'll do that from time to time," I say in a deadpan.

"Damn nearly went off the chart. Thought I'd find you dead in here."

"In a sense, I have died." If she broaches the subject, I am thinking, I will cite Woody Allen: Don't knock masturbation. It's sex with someone I love.

I see an expression of compunction in her eyes, as she thinks she has strayed into sensitive territory having mentioned death.

"You're going to do great tomorrow, Bob. Really. Dr. Morrow developed the procedure himself. You couldn't have a better surgeon."

"Thanks," I say. "You know, I think I'd like to be alone."

That night Samuel Cohen, our family rabbi, shows up with Mom and Dad, who are now separated. Richard has sent his wishes and fears with them, and is sorry he couldn't be here. He has recently returned from Israel where he had gone to take a measure of solace in his faith, the faith of our ancestors. Laurie won't arrive from New Jersey until after my surgery. So in the meantime, our four voices mix as we relive our family's shared past, our uneven history as observant Jews and not-so-terribly-observant Jews. Rabbi Cohen finds an uncanny humor and poignancy in our history, perhaps because he knows it so well. He knows of my mother's death, of the marriage that promptly followed, of the savage impact of IHSS on our clan. He is a Canadian and speaks like one, enunciating each syllable of every word impeccably, using the spoken word with a strange fastidiousness. This aspect of his character is reflected in the theatrical elegance of his dress and the pipe he keeps cocked in the corner of his mouth, the slender stem swooping like a swan's neck to the bowl.

Soon the family leaves and Rabbi Cohen and I are left alone. An awkward silence settles between us, ushering in the murky sounds of the hospital beyond the door. I observe his bowed figure while waiting for him to speak.

"So, Bob, are you frightened?" he finally asks.

"Sometimes I'm terrified, other times I'm not whatsoever."

"Would it help to talk about this fear?"

"You know what would help?"

"What's that?"

"Would you mind taking me up to the chapel?"

We are sitting in the half-light on a miniature pew, my voice sullen, almost melancholy. I am telling him how my thoughts have continually returned to my mother lately, how I haven't really thought of her in any meaningful way until now. I share with him the image I have salvaged: the posture of the wheelchair, her weak hand poised in the air, waving goodbye to her sons. *Blood of my blood, flesh of my flesh, memory of my memory.* I ask him to ask the god of Abraham, Isaac, and Jacob to have my mother watch over me. I feel tears rising up as I tell Rabbi Cohen, "This disease—this is what she lived and died by."

Looking back upon that dim-lit room with its slightly miniature design, its air of having seen so much grief and absorbing so many sobbed prayers, the sense you had of being so high above it all on the top floor, I now understand how close I was to my mother then. The boundaries between her and me were dissolved, and those between Richard and me as well. For that brief moment the three of us inhabited one trembling body.

. . .

Not long after awakening the following morning I am visited by a Red Cross volunteer, a pretty woman in her late fifties, silver hair, dignified in her speech and manner. She approaches my bed, smiling, the little Red Cross emblem floating over her heart, and asks if I am Robert Pensack.

"Unfortunately, I am Robert Pensack today."

She grimaces sympathetically at the remark. "I understand you have IHSS?"

"That's right. And I'm due in the OR in an hour."

"We see a lot of the disease here."

"So you know what it is?"

"Oh, yes. And I know that Dr. Morrow has had a lot of success with your operation."

"He developed the procedure, isn't that correct?"

"That's right." She pauses. Her eyes drift toward the window and she says with an unambiguous tenderness, "You know, there are worse diseases than IHSS. What I mean to say is that at least they have a treatment for it. We see a lot of people for whom we can do nothing."

"I've seen a few of them. I keep telling myself I am a lucky young man."

She smiles expansively, then tells me I'll be in her thoughts and prayers. But just as she is about to turn and head out the door, I notice her small name tag with MRS. MORROW discreetly stamped into the brass.

"You wouldn't happen to be related to Dr. Morrow, would you?"

"Yes. He's my husband."

"I see."

She then comes to my bedside, kisses my forehead, and leaves.

A few minutes later my parents file into the room bearing small gifts and cards. As we exchange small talk my thoughts drift to Richard and how his eyes would be displaying concealed pain if he were here. He never expected his little brother to go under the knife first. At some level I think he feels more comfortable being the pioneer, playing the role of Big Brother, then preparing me for what's in store. That role comes more naturally to him. But now here I am, lying on my back, a sky-blue nightgown covering a chest that is about to be parted, a heart that will be stopped, cut into, then sewn back together. I see now how this picture would hurt him. He would understand this is his future too.

Half an hour later two orderlies appear from behind Mom and Dad, a little hurried and anxious to get down to business. My parents back away to allow for the gurney, and I hoist myself onto the starched white sheets, calm, joking. With little ado they quickly wheel me out the door and round the corner with my parents following, their talk focused on anything but the surgery. My dad escorts the gurney, his voice constant at my side, telling me to stay calm, everything will be all right, the voice rolling down the hall to the steady ictus of the squeaking wheels, all the way to the wooden swinging doors of the OR. His voice is there then is suddenly gone. I feel the inexorable progress of the gurney, the panic of being trapped, the knowledge that there is nothing I can do to escape this body, the loss of control. In the operating room the anesthesiologist greets me from behind a blue mask then lifts the glasses from my face, and I lose myself in foggy vision. There is the dominant whiteness of the surgical light and faceless voices, the anesthesiologist talking to me as he slides a needle into my forearm, then there is Dr. Morrow. He asks me how I feel and I hear myself say fine, just fine, and a translucent mask is lowered over the mouth followed by the sensation of claustrophobia, loss of breath. I am told to count backwards but I don't even try as I struggle against the anesthesia. Then there is nothing. Only a world of shadows.

20

Because it is stronger than you are, do not struggle against it; become supplicant, ease your way through the world of reflective surfaces, allow the respirator to govern your breath. Because of the scene that awaits you, it is best to drift back into the morphine sleep, let your mind dissolve into the shadowy underworld where nothing is at stake.

My eyelids flutter apart and the view ruthlessly presents itself. Sunlight bleeds through blue curtains, shallow waves of noise float through the cubicle, upon my chest I see a large plastic box with flashing lights which suggest to my softened mind that I am part machine, part flesh and blood. My eyes roam across the blue of the curtains, I gasp for breath against the absolute will of the respirator, my stomach fills with air, then I am submerged into dreamless sleep.

Perhaps it is the mutation of time or the convective cycle of sleep and wakefulness, but what seems to be but a breath later I am alert, my eyes absorbing the blue curtains saturated with sunlight, the noises all about me, and what I recognize to be an external pacemaker that sits atop my chest like a small robot syncopating the beat of my heart. I know the machine from scrubbing in on heart surgery last summer while working for Dr. Steele, and now here it is, a part of me, the bionics of the Tin

Man. The nurse, Maria, notices my fluttering eyelids and she wipes my brow with a terry cloth towel. I try to ask, Why the pacemaker? but can't move. She immediately begins imploring me to relax, that I'm on a respirator and that's why I can't talk. It will be a few days, so just go back to sleep, I'll be happier, really I will. I want to tell her my stomach is distended, bloated with air, but she doesn't comprehend.

A few minutes later my dad and Dr. Morrow enter the room. Dad asks why I appear so agitated, and Dr. Morrow tells him I'm probably just scared, overwhelmed by the scene. I gesture to my dad as I thrash about that I want a pen and paper, and he asks Maria, who gives him a small pad and a pen clipped to her breast pocket. With my shaking left hand I write on the tiny pink pad an inscrutable message: *Belly bloated!* Maria immediately produces a nasogastric tube from a drawer, then inserts it into a nostril and down into the esophagus where it finally breaches the esophageal sphincter. The air is released, there is instant and total relief and my dad's eyes smile. Slowly, very slowly at first, I drift off to sleep, awaking every now and then to see my hand in my father's, his soft voice filling the cubicle of curtains with questions for Dr. Morrow and Maria.

A few days later, with the endotracheal tube of the respirator wedged into the top of my windpipe, Dr. Morrow and Dad enter the room. My father seats himself on a corner of the mattress next to my shoulder, his posture attentively erect, as Dr. Morrow situates himself at the perimeter of curtains, poised to address us as father and son.

"You're still experiencing a little heart failure, Bob, and that's why we still have you on the respirator, but you'll be off tomorrow," he begins, his voice vaguely apologetic. He holds his hands clasped behind him. "I see you've learned not to fight against it."

I nod and manage a weak smile. Dad sits quiet and thoughtful at my side.

"We had a little difficulty in the OR, though. I know you used to be an athlete, and I know that one of your hopes for this operation was to be able to participate in sports once again. What I mean to say is that I was a little too . . . zealous in thinning the septal wall and inadvertently put a small tear, or hole in it."

I feel my eyelids flutter, butterfly kisses to the sky.

He widens his stance, rolling his weight forward on the balls of his small feet. His eyes are fixed on mine, glazed and reddened with an expression of deep hurt like those of a small child.

"But you fixed that and now he's as good as new," my father abruptly says to Dr. Morrow to occupy the silence.

"Well, what we did was open up the right ventricle and sew in a Dacron patch over the hole. But unfortunately the hole damaged the heart's natural electrical conduction system; the pacemaker tissue was injured.* That explains the external pacemaker sitting on your chest." He points to the box then emphasizes, "It's temporary, however. We're pretty confident that your heart will recover and a pacemaker won't be necessary."

"That's right," my dad says, patting the whitened tendons of my hand. "Unnecessary."

"Bob . . . I'm sorry." His head is bowed slightly as though in an attempt to cloak any display of grief. "But hopefully these complications won't affect your long-term recovery."

He goes on to explain the structure of the heart, the basics of electrical conduction through the muscle, the arcane nature of the pacing process. When he's finished he asks if I have any questions, offering me pen and paper, and I wave my head that I un-

---

*The human heart is an electrical-mechanical pump. Every beat is initiated first by an electrical impulse that begins in the heart's specialized pacemaker system, which travels through the septum.

derstand while trying to fight off the impulse to cry, as it would counter the rhythm of the respirator. I lie back mute, blinking, inert. His explanations are all familiar to me.

My dad stands as the meeting comes to a natural close and kisses my cheek before leaving, then Dr. Morrow comes to my side, places a hand on my shoulder, and whispers, "I'm sorry, Bob." I see the lines cutting into the forehead, the fragmented pattern that has worked its way into his cheeks seemingly overnight. When he leaves the room goes quiet. I stare up into the pattern of the hanging ceiling, my mind frozen, dwelling on the syncopated wheezing and the pools of light of the pacemaker. Finally the thunder of my wounded heart fills my ears.

Years later I will happen upon a shocking revelation, a story that will alter my sensibilities. Although I never confirmed this, during a checkup at the NIH, I will discover that Dr. Morrow himself has suffered from the symptoms of IHSS almost all his adult life, and a relative of his happened to be having a pacemaker implanted at the time of my visit.

The days flutter by, and just as he had expected my heart begins to recover, keeping its own pace most of the time without the assistance of the pacemaker which, I have been told, only kicks in upon sensing that the heart is failing at the task of keeping cadence. The respirator is removed five days postsurgery, allowing my lungs to work under their own volition. Eventually I'm allowed to stand and walk about the room, then the following day I manage to shuffle my way down to the solarium to visit with the other heart patients. When I arrive I am taken in like lost family; nearly everyone here has recently had surgery and shuffles around with me with the same posture that suggests the general lumbar pain of geriatric patients. We all grip our IV poles and indiscreetly groan as our chests haven't healed. We wear bathrobes and slippers, and appear profoundly shaken. The scene strikes me as touching and pathetic, grimly humorous; I mutter over the voices and groaning and squeaking of the IV wheels, "Hey, everybody, let's do the Boogaloo," and there is shocked laughter followed by more groaning. The fresh incisions and healing of breastbone don't allow for mirth.

As we move about in a perfunctory pattern through the solarium, I see a five-year-old Greek boy whom I recognize from the days prior to the surgery. He hobbles his way down the hall like an elderly dwarf, dragging along his IV pole, careful of his chest wound, his eyes flat and harrowed. I vaguely recall his congenital heart defect, the family's story of coming to the United States for help, and now here they are, the parents with their hands to their cheeks, each flanking his progress on either side as he approaches. As I make my way toward him, his head lifts, smiling, shirking off pain, careful of any movement from the waist up. He groans "Hello," then his parents come to my side and ask my name in very broken English.

"Bob Pensack," I say, carefully enunciating each syllable. "I'm from Colorado."

"That's him," they whisper to one another with happy astonishment. They are a handsome couple, almost twinlike in their manners, their jet-black hair and rich dark skin. The similar cadence of their voices lends a musical quality to their adopted language. After a breathless pause the mother finally speaks, as her English seems to be the more sophisticated of the two.

"We understand you are a medical student." They stare at me admiringly, waiting for my response.

"That's right," I say. "This operation is part of my training. I go to a school that requires unusual dedication."

For a moment they believe absolutely what I just said. They gaze at each other, beautiful and innocent as deer, their eyes growing ineffable, and they repeat in tandem with their brown eyes fixed on the other's ". . . part of my training," then they simultaneously break out in hard laughter. The boy and I gaze at one another then try to laugh softly without inflating our lungs.

"I understand. A joke," the husband says as the lingering echoes of laughter scatter through the web of corridors.

A moment later I look down at the boy and see he has grown sullen. He lifts a small closed hand to his mouth and gently coughs which causes him to wince. I set a hand on his soft black hair and he looks up and tries to say something in English.

"What's that?" I ask.

He repeats it then waves his hand, indicating it hurts to speak.

"That's all right," I say, feeling a fresh assault of tears. The sudden wave of emotion startles me. Trying not to sound maudlin, I add with a shaky voice, "We're all going to get better."

As the weeks pass, the heart seems to heal itself. It grows stronger, knitting together its flesh where it had been cut, like a broken bone that has set. Eventually the doctors remove the pacemaker leads and the heart proves to be capable of prodding itself with its own silent flicker of electricity just as Dr. Morrow had predicted. Gradually there is talk of being discharged.

Then one morning, one of my first since having been disconnected from the battery of monitors, I am examined by two nurses before being sent on my way to the echocardiogram lab where they will take a two-dimensional picture of the inside of my heart using sound waves. This morning, however, I am feeling a little light-headed, and though I've made the trip before, I ask if I may have one of them accompany me.

"You'll be all right, Bob. Really," the heavier-set of the two says with a matronly manner.

"I just don't feel entirely normal."

"You've walked there before. It's time to start trusting your heart a little, Bob."

"Really, I'm not feeling at all well . . ."

Without a word the other nurse checks my pulse. Her cool fingers sink against my carotid artery, her eyes freeze to the face of her wristwatch. A quiet moment passes and she says I'm fine, that I have nothing to worry about.

"It's common for heart patients to feel a little anxious and unsure of themselves just prior to being discharged," she says. Her voice is a whisper.

The heavier nurse agrees. "It's normal," she says, shrugging her round shoulders.

"I'm telling you I don't *feel* normal . . ."

She throws her hands up and rolls her large eyes in resignation.

"All right all right all right." She steps out from behind the nurses' station and escorts me down the hall, talking all the way. Her accent is Bronx and very harsh. As I trudge along I gradually sense her voice becoming part of the background, a gnawing white noise; my head grows heavy, then a moment later I swoon. The beat of my heart comes to the fore, the slow stammer, the diminishing pulse loud in my ears. The nurse continues to jabber while I feel my heart limping in my chest. The mind fades as its source of bright-red blood slows and slows to a trickle. "My heart's stopping! It's stopping!" Then I hear the nurse's voice cease in midsentence, and she turns to me, a small hand covering the dark circle of her mouth. She yells for Dr. Borer, a cardiologist, who comes sprinting down the hall. My eyes blink, the eyelashes flutter like insect wings as Dr. Borer quickly places the electrocardiogram leads on my chest. I feel my heart is about to come to an abrupt halt. At first there is terror, twirling colors, overwhelming claustrophobia, but I sense myself moving beyond that, beyond what I recognize as the phenomenal world into a peaceful country of shadows, an incomprehensible realm of sublime calm. The body—my body—floats, and as it does so I experience the ability to observe myself, the doctors and nurses in the laboratory where the electrocardiogram ushers out a ribbon of white paper with a steady black line from its mouth. The staff gleam as they briskly move about in their white coats in this vacuum of time. From above I witness the life drift from the body, feel the Self separate into its component parts. Yet there is no panic. Only light and calm. Observing my own death I am impassive. This is the only surprise, and yet it is no surprise at all.

I visualize Dr. Borer beating away at my chest, the arched spine beneath the white coat and the straight line bifurcating the tape. Then it wavers, gently at first, then radically, and whatever it is that binds body to spirit, that substanceless primordial stuff, pulls me back; there is sensation, phenomena, what we recognize as experience.

Then I look up into the concerned and shocked face of Dr. Borer, my eyelids batting away the light. My head flops to the side, rotating upon the limp neck, and I see a pile of tape pouring forth from the electrocardiogram, a terrifying document, a heap of meaningless confetti. Then I begin to quiver and cry as all I see about me is the unbearable terror of this world, the immense burden of being alive.

21

That afternoon I am taken to surgery where a permanent pace-maker is implanted into my abdomen just to the left of the belly button. It is the size and shape of a tin of snuff, suspended just under the skin like a can of Skoal in the hip pocket of a pair of tight jeans. I learn that the damaged electrical system of my heart has revealed itself as being, in the words of Dr. Borer, undependable.

For the next few days I sense I've changed. My hands shake, my concentration is nonexistent, a pile of magazines sits neat and dusty on the nightstand as I lie wakeful and alert through a wilderness of sights and sounds. There is sensory stimuli and a network of raw nerves at the mercy of a chaotic universe with no order, no security. Questions arise, both medical and ontological, having to do with my sanity and the nature of this terrible new awareness. The mind doesn't work with the familiar pattern that it did just a few weeks ago. At times I become strangely detached from the environment, particularly in the midst of loud noises or multiple conversations. I am accosted by the everyday, overwhelmed by the mundane. And the symptoms are terrifying; I break out in a hot sweat, become dizzy with the secret but powerful secretion of adrenaline, my mind boils with disparate thoughts as the world transforms itself into an elaborate disaster. All I know is that I am naked and alive. During the brief stretches of calm I attempt to ponder my condition, and slowly it

occurs to me that these symptoms could represent some subtle
brain damage incurred during the surgery. But mere explanations of course provide no relief, because all I now know is that I
am deeply and irrevocably out of my mind.

Within three or four days I am given permission to leave the
hospital for lunch with my father. Earlier in the day he called to
say he would pick me up at the front door at noon, so I have
spent the morning preparing myself for what I expect to be a
perilous foray into the world of sharp edges and random vio-
lence. So now, as I approach the sun-brightened doors at the end
of the corridor, I at once try with meager strength to hobble this
fragile body into the sunlight and keep the mind balanced and
rational.

Outside, beyond the rich orange and red leaves of a maple,
beyond the stillness and darkness of the hospital corridor,
beyond the gray wedge of the sidewalk, my father's black
Porsche 911-S Targa squats like a panther against the curb. I
lean into the glass door, carefully feeling it give way to a wild
swirl of dry autumn air, then feel the impact of sunlight against
skin. The warmth is ancient, a memory of another life. I see the
door to the Targa ease open and my father step out from within
its low feline posture, smiling with pride. But I hardly notice
him. The autumn setting astonishes the senses, the pores of skin
are flooded with warmth, the Indian summer ripe with color. In
the small gardens straddling the sidewalk are the opaque crests
of tulip bulbs, toward the street sit two ripe gourds carved into
jack-o'-lanterns. A cloud of sparrows descends and pecks at the
seed scattered on the lawn. As I watch the simple scene arrange
itself, I feel the intense warmth of sunlight upon my face followed by an inscrutable rush of tears compressing in my eyes. I
can't help myself. After a brief rest I walk on toward the car into
my father's outstretched arms, then work my way into the false
security of his new sports car. We sit for a moment in silence,

listening to the precision of the idling engine, waiting for the
tears to ebb. He asks if I'm all right and I tell him that I think so;
he then puts the car in gear and we fade into the violent confusion of city traffic. Within a few minutes I am filling the car
with cries for my father to slow down, to be more careful; he
looks over at his deranged wide-eyed son who keeps a hand
braced against the dash, his face sweating, vigilant of every car
passed as the Porsche rolls down a shady brick avenue.

After a full five weeks spent within the small rooms and halls of
Building 10 of the NIH, I leave for my parents' house in New
Jersey to convalesce. As grand pawn in the divorce settlement, it
stands uninhabited with a realtor's sign driven into the immaculate brown lawn. A friend of mine from college, "Bahama" Bob
Korn, comes to stay with me and nurses this broken body back
to health. He is an immense and gentle man, slightly effeminate
in his manner, unemployed and very eccentric in touching ways.
As a private nurse he is magnificent with his utter lack of
squeamishness and his ability to suppress any revulsion in what
he sees. He also possesses an authentic willingness to be at my
disposal through the long days during which he shares with me
what's on his convoluted mind. I lie back captivated by his im-
passioned soliloquies, amazed at this large man's selflessness.

One day, one of my first full days home, I feel an uneasy curi-
osity coming to bear. While Bahama is in the kitchen fixing
lunch for us, I slip into my parents' former bedroom and stand
naked to the waist before a full-length mirror, taking in the
scars, the bulge of the pacemaker, the disfigured breastbone. I
hear myself gasp, an audible breath of shock. Then I don't move
or make any sound; the distant clamor of Bahama working in the
kitchen fades and the pounding of my heart fills my ears. I stand
before the mirror mesmerized, horrified, full of the disbelief that

what I am observing is a reflection of my body, a picture of my own flesh and bone. I stare closely at the misshapen contours of the pacemaker, the crescent incisional scar, then the T-scar where I observe the barely perceptible pulse of my heart against my wounded chest. All sounds die, I mouth the words, *I am twenty-five years old.* My hands and feet tingle as I run my fingers along the purple seams. For what must be fifteen minutes I stand there, lost in the history of wounds, then Bahama approaches me from behind, quiet, his voice soft.

"Come on, Bob," he says, placing his warm hands on my shoulders and steering me away from the mirror. "Our lunch is getting cold."

In the silence a teakettle can be heard shrieking in the kitchen.

While sitting at the table before bowls of stew and club sandwiches, Bahama gradually becomes animated as he tells fantastic stories. Soon he has me laughing with a hand to my chest. During a pause in one of his narratives I tell him that I'm thinking of having something made, a swimsuit of the 1920s or 1930s vintage, the kind that is made with a top. It would be something I'd wear at the reservoir next summer when I take Allison swimming.

"Why would you want something like that?" he asks.

"Why do you think?"

"Well, to hide your scars, but . . ." he says meekly.

"But what?"

"Well, nothing."

So later that afternoon he drives me down to a tailor. Again I am terrified by what I interpret as reckless driving on the part of Bahama. He gradually slows the car to a crawl, every now and then glancing over at my pale face and the sheen of tiny sweat droplets around my mouth and forehead. He is stunned and probably a little hurt by my behavior. After the twenty-minute drive we arrive at the tailor, both of us silent. Once I've recovered I apologize and try to explain my new fears. "Oh, no, no, no. Don't apologize. I understand, I understand," he says, laying a long thick arm across my back.

The tailor, as it turns out, is outrageously flamboyant—his gestures wide, his voice simpering and arrogant, his wavy hair beyond the realm of chic. I describe to him what I want and he listens very attentively and grows more and more excited as the description becomes complete. I don't explain that I have a chest of disfiguring scars, or that I am twenty-five years old and over-whelmed with adolescent insecurities concerning my body. Nor do I explain that I have a girlfriend waiting for me in Denver. But the tailor simply sees it as a passionate fashion statement, something for which he has boundless enthusiasm. Bahama stands back, just beyond the tailor's field of view as he inspects a rack of suitcoats, trying to squelch his laughter. The tailor winces and softly bites with relish into a knuckle as sublime images reveal themselves to his raging imagination.

"This is an absolutely delicious idea," he says.

"Well, I want it kept pretty plain, nothing too . . . baroque," I say, struggling for a more neutral synonym for flowery.

Lightly clapping both hands together, he says, "I know *exactly* what to do with this . . . gem. That's what this idea is, you know. It's an absolute gem."

Bahama drives slowly and deliberately home. He makes innuendos about my stoicism while being measured and mockingly reassures me that the tailor will come up with exactly what I had in mind, something I'll wear all the time, on the beach and off.

"Well, you sure went to the right place, eh?" he says.

"I think he'll do a pretty good job."

"He'll do a great job, it'll be absolutely smashing." He manfully pats my knee.

After two weeks under Bahama's care, I feel I'm becoming physically ready to make the flight back to Denver. The day before my departure I receive a phone call from the tailor saying his "little project" is complete. So that afternoon I head down to the shop, this time driving myself. I am very excited and hopeful. What I want to be reassured of is that I can look and act like everyone else, even if it means dressing a little differently, that all will be as it once was. But when I enter the shop, the tailor solemnly comes at me with what he has come up with, not speaking, not even smiling, his arms theatrically presenting his creation of lace and frills, expecting me to be dumbfounded with awe. I try to muster composure.

"I've been dying for you to come back," he says with utmost seriousness. There is a long dramatic pause. "Isn't it something? Here, I want you to try it on." He holds the acrylic fabric to my chest, eyes me up and down.

So I go to the dressing room, cursing under my breath, trying to be polite. I carefully ease out of my street clothes and pull on the tailor's creation and see that my back is exposed as one would expect in a woman's suit. Looking at myself in the mirror I see a clown, a disfigured sexless clown. Beneath the red and blue stretch fabric I can make out the faint outline of the pacemaker. The front is cut so low, explicitly low really, that the peak of the T-scar shows; just to the right I see the cadence of my heart, the steady ticking against my sternum. Standing in the cold and quiet I feel another abrupt wave of tears as I am convinced I can't return to Denver like this. I turn away from the mirror, then the tears come all at once and I turn back to the reflection one last time to take in the ridiculous figure. For that one moment I absorb all the despair, all the agony and condense it into a singular image of myself in this outrageous getup. Then there is a sudden unexpected burst of laughter. I walk out from behind the curtain where the tailor stands looking puzzled by both my glistening face and what he takes to be a stunning sight. He holds his palms pressed together as in prayer, fingertips covering the arch of his nose and slowly closes his eyes as though savoring an image of a deity.

"This is absolutely gorgeous," he says, walking in a loose circle around me like a barber. He inspects his work, fussing with the straps then with the hem of his trunks. Eventually he stands, sympathetically and candidly looking me in the eye, and says, "It made you cry, didn't it?" He smiles with the certainty he has read my mind. "It's so magnificent it made you cry."

"It did."

"So the materials were ten dollars and the labor was forty. So that comes to fifty all added up."

Either out of some deep and nocturnal fascination for the absurd, for camp, or simply to mock this ridiculous body, I say with hearty conviction: "It's gorgeous."

22

As I emerge from the pressurized cabin along with a weary stream of passengers and step onto the concourse, I see the familiar faces as in a dream—smiling, pasty-white, vigorous, congratulatory, uncomprehending. I glide across the carpet feeling my feet vanish beneath me. Then I see the signs dancing in the air: WELCOME HOME, BOB! and suddenly sense the spirit slip from my body. I observe myself in much the same way as I had in the echo-lab. Within a few phantom steps I am swallowed by the crowd and taken into the rowdy arms of friends then delivered through a tunnel of bodies to Allison. She stands with her arms folded, smiling wryly, her hair pulled up into the familiar buoyant ponytail. I am ineluctably ushered before her like a pagan sacrifice to the altar. The atmosphere grows quiet as she stares at me as though I've been a bad boy.

"Hello, Bob," she says.

This produces a chorus of hoots, catcalls.

"Nice to see you, Allison," I say. My voice sounds removed. She then takes me into her arms, and all hell breaks loose.

I am sitting in the lecture hall, the panorama of the periodical chart, the tops of heads, the airy vastness of the room twirling in my field of view. My moistened hand cramps as it struggles to grip the shaking pen. I keep telling myself that if I can just hold on everything will drift back to normal. To my left I hear Allison's pen rushing across page after page, gleaning the pertinent information from the lecture. Meanwhile, my hand lies crippled, gripped with palsy. My mind roams through the collage of traumatic history, unable to focus on the lesson while the heart pulsates in my ears. *My heart has a hole in it, I have suffered my first cardiac arrest. I am twenty-five years old and want to become a doctor.* At the end of the lecture there is the clap of books being closed, the rustle of papers, the high-pitched whine of backpacks being zipped closed. Allison collects her things beside me and turns in shock at my sweaty shaky profile. Then she looks down at my empty page, the two inscrutable lines of notes just beneath the date.

"Oh my god, Bob," she whispers.

Our eyes meet in horror.

"Something's wrong with my mind, Allison."

For the next few days I manage to leave my apartment promptly every morning at eight and head to lecture then to lab. I am more than six weeks behind my medical school class and since my return I haven't retained a thing. Slowly it becomes clear this is all a charade. In the mornings I feel more or less normal, but once away from the shelter of the apartment I am attacked by the hostile blue sky, the anger of the December wind, the flurry of traffic. What is most startling is that everyone around me appears oblivious to danger. They go about their business unaware of the fragility of the human organism, naively assuming the shadow of death is stalking everyone but them. I am terrified and amazed. But who am I other than an ordinary madman; I know that I have changed, that this new awareness is not normal, and at the same time I am convinced this is the elemental structure of the universe. As R. D. Laing once asserted, one wonders whether the schizophrenic's perspective is distorted or whether they are more acutely in tune with the absurd nature of reality.

A week later I stand shoulder-to-shoulder with classmates in a surgery suite as we are about to observe a simple rib resection. The patient's chest X rays hang before a light board, the haunting gray picture displaying the growth of an opaque tumor bulging like an onion bulb from the sixth rib. As we all stand before the anesthetized patient reposed upon the table, I feel the grip of a deep panic. My face floods the sky-blue mask with perspiration as I witness the scalpel glide through the flesh. The skin parts, revealing in the wake of the knife the sugary veined muscle and pouches of cutaneous fat. I look about at my classmates, their eyes dull and undaunted like those of cattle, unmoved by the trauma they are witnessing. The anonymous expressions above the masks follow the bloody trail with a detachment that I now understand to be far beyond me. When it comes time to remove the tumorous section of rib, the surgeon asks the nurse for the surgical coping saw with which he resects it. All the while my classmates look on, now becoming animated as their fascination heightens, proud as I once was of possessing the ability to observe flesh and blood without so much as a wince. Unlike me they do not identify themselves with patients and corpses but with the immortal surgeon. Soon the soft grating of the saw becomes intolerable. I indiscreetly excuse myself and head directly for the men's room where mental pictures dominate my imagination as I stand before the mirror. I see the knife sinking into my side, the saw coming to bear. I feel all the cold and sharpness of the scalpel descending into the lean flesh while I remind myself that I am not the patient. I am here, safe and alive, a simple medical student. Safe and alive. I tell myself I have blurred my boundaries, that all the pain of this world is not necessarily my pain. What I have lost is that simple emotional mechanism that allows the human mind to divorce itself from the imagination so that it may work deliberately. Apparently now I am overwhelmed by its terrifying power.

As the weeks pass I withdraw more and more into my apartment. Every morning I close the door behind me to the peace and quiet of the apartment with my backpack slung over my shoulder and venture out into the open air, into the wide-open spaces shared by perfect strangers. Then I sense I am at the mercy of the elements. After a few blocks I become dizzy and terrified and hobble back as best I can to the safety of the apartment. After two weeks of this, I become housebound, holed-up like a troll in my dark and quiet room.

Friends come around asking questions, the sheer solicitude distorting their faces and voices above the brass door-chain. I tell them I'm not feeling well, that I am experiencing some mild complications from the surgery, and after a set of probing questions they leave, unsatisfied and puzzled. Only Allison is aware of the nature of my problems, and even she is baffled and put off by the altered personality. A mere month ago I was a convivial and bright medical student. Now I'm a frightened and insane recluse. Her appearances at my door become infrequent as the symptoms intensify and I withdraw. Soon they cease altogether.

And so my depression compounds itself as I come to understand that I am losing everything that I have ever valued. It becomes clear that I have dropped out of school, that becoming a doctor is now a pipe dream, that I will never heal myself. My girlfriend has left me, and my body will forever be a source of deep shame. This is to be a life in which I will never participate.

Then one night as I sit in the vacuum of darkness and silence, watching the accumulation of large dry snowflakes over the city, I feel the nearing of panic. As I stand before my own ghostly reflection in the glass it occurs to me that I haven't left my apartment all day. Then slowly, like an apparition, the symptoms return; there is the general sense of removal, the grainy texture of a soundless movie, the colors like those of a sepiatone. I think of those ancient photographs of dead relatives on my father's nightstand. Their eyes gazed back almost expressionless, as though they were remembering us, not us remembering them. The haunted legacy. The room suddenly expands, the walls rush away, a chill settles over the apartment. I flashback to my recent resuscitation and step before the full-length mirror where I run my eyes over the geography of scars. The soft thud builds in my ears as I stand there, and gradually subdues all the other small sounds of the apartment. I take a chair and set it before the mirror then observe the subtle tap of the bloody invisible muscle against the breastbone. Fractions of hours and hours pass within the steady drum in my ears, and slowly the terror swells. Everything is gone, I say aloud. Then I see myself quivering in the mirror, and there is the immense certainty of impending doom. On the shelf beside the mirror I take up a sheathed Bowie knife and carefully slide it from the soft leather. A peculiar mental dialogue develops in which I ask myself if I am willing to watch my courage dissolve in my hands. All the while I gaze back at my chest where the insults of this heart express themselves. The integrity of the body has been altered beyond the grace of nature, I think to myself, and now— I run the cool blade over the woody texture of scars, watching its progress in the mirror. Then directly over the visible pulse it halts. I tell myself the only thing left to do is to stab this alien heart, pop it like a big red balloon. If I truly want to avenge my mother's death and Richard's and my impending deaths, then what I should do now is sink this tiny dagger into the source of the degradation. From the glinting tip of the knife pours a faint trickle of blood that forms a pool in the impress. I pull the knife away and poise it a few inches from the pulse. I tell myself this would be the ultimate act of bravery, to stab this treasonous heart through and through until it can no longer beat. Then I look myself in the eye in the mirror, losing myself in my own gaze. I slowly lower the knife, drawing it away from the chest and lay it on the floor. Once the knife leaves my hand I begin to cry like I never have before. I realize I am trapped in this body, that I can't go on and that I must go on. This is the nature of being. This is the soul of this terrible new awareness.

The following morning I leave the apartment, frightened and vigilant, and drive to Allison's apartment. When I arrive she stands in the doorway, deeply shocked, almost frightened by my appearance. I try to act normal, as though nothing has ever been wrong, but the act merely strikes her as bizarre and disturbing.

"So how's class been going, Allison?" I ask, my mouth twitching from nerves.

"Fine, Bob. I assume you haven't left your apartment in a while?"

"Oh, no, I leave it all the time. I'm hardly there, actually."

This banter keeps up for several minutes, and she asks finally if I want a drink, which I decline. She walks off to the kitchen to fix herself one. As she talks to me from beyond the hanging cabinets and Formica counter, I walk over to the sliding glass doors and step out onto the balcony. The sun is strong as it reflects off the bright new snow. From outside I catch Allison's muffled voice, distorted by distance, the slightly opened door, and the vortex of my own swirling mind. I hear the jingle of ice cubes, the shifting of bottles over the counter, and meanwhile I gaze over the balustrade and stare into the thin fabric of snow covering the frozen earth six stories below. Soon my mind is dismissing all the other sounds and sensations and I am gripped by my suicidal imagination. I ask myself what it would be like to fall, the sensation of succumbing to the earth, the irresistible pull of gravity, the pain and then the absence of pain as my skull collided with the continent. Abominable questions. After an uncertain passing of time, I feel a hand on my shoulder, and turn to see Allison's horrified face. At once she understands where my mind has been.

"I need help," I say, just before breaking down.

"I think so."

I walk back into the apartment, slowly and decisively, my body quivering with fear.

"What should I do?" I ask.

"What any good physician would."

I sit myself down on the sofa and try to bring my breathing under control and shirk this feeling of portent. At last I grasp some semblance of concentration and try to observe my behavior with a certain detachment. Aloud I say, "What am I doing here?"

Allison stares sympathetically at my hunched figure. "For a minute there I thought you forgot we have a staircase."

"I did," I say without turning to her. Peripherally I see her looking down at the floor.

"You need to make a phone call, Bob."

"Right."

Allison sifts through the limber bulk of the Denver white pages and writes down the number for the University of Colorado Hospital psychiatric emergency room. When I call, a woman's voice on the other end asks a series of exasperating questions such as my name and address, and for a moment I feel this isn't the answer. Suddenly I am panicked. "What I need now," I tell her, "is relief from these symptoms." "I understand, Robert. This will only take a moment." Soon she has a psychiatrist on the phone, a man with a barely audible voice by the name of Dr. Jay Scully. After describing my condition, he asks if I could come down to the emergency room, and I tell him absolutely yes.

I arrive at the hospital a few minutes later shaking and nervous, but hopeful, something I haven't felt for several weeks now. The anticipation of relief itself brings relief. The receptionist immediately escorts me to Dr. Scully's office down a long dark hall where he sits behind a small desk mulling over a field of papers. When he stands to introduce himself I am stunned by his sheer physical size. He stands six and a half feet tall and weighs well over two hundred seventy-five pounds; it occurs to me that he tries to diminish his physical mass with this tiny soft voice, which is like that of an excruciatingly shy but oversized child. He offers me a seat with a timid gesture of his long arm, and he begins with a gentle interrogation. I reply by telling him as much as I can about myself within an hour: the surgery, the hole in my heart, the cardiac arrest, and finally this deadly terror. The exchange strikes me as strange, almost burlesque in nature; here sits a man nearly twice my size behind a miniature desk listening with an intensity I have never before witnessed, who speaks so softly his voice is barely audible at all. However, I instantly feel safe and experience a momentary reprieve from what has been constant terror. An uninterrupted hour passes without his whispering more than fifty words, and he finally tells me that I should definitely seek the help of a psychiatrist, and that he thinks I'll get better if I do so. Then he tells me I'll be referred to another psychiatrist, a Dr. Ted Gaensbauer. For a moment I feel the floor give way, finding the mere presence of this man to be soothing in itself. He obviously senses my letdown and explains that Dr. Gaensbauer is assigned to medical-student mental-health patients. Dr. Scully then scribbles on a notepad a prescription for Librium, a mild tranquilizer which he says will diminish the severity of the anxiety. Just as the brief session comes to an end, he hands me the slip of paper as a meager offering, then tells me to hang in there, help is on its way.

23

The library houses an air of solemnity. Here I feel safe from the echo of whispers, crowds and faces, the suffocation of etiquette. With the ease of a child I can inhabit the endless corridors of books, the study carrels, the sofas tucked in corners. It is here I invest most of my day. I digest all the psychiatric, neurological and cardiac literature that may apply to my condition. I begin with medical texts which eventually refer me to bibliographies on specific symptoms similar to mine. Taking the names of specialists I move on to the periodical department of the library which provides the very latest thought and technology. Again and again the same names keep coming up. At first I focus on emotional disorders simply because the symptoms are far and away the most lethal. But it quickly becomes clear that this tactic is naive. My heart and mind are too intimately damaged, the past they share too common, and what I glean from the days and nights of study is the intuitive belief that there is something larger at work here, something that connects all the elements of my broken mind and body. But I only have a faint clue of what it is, a silhouette guiding me through fog.

So the days in the library become fluid, mornings blending into evenings unnoticed. Occasionally I'll glance at the sheet of thermal windows toward the east end of the library to learn whether it's time to sleep or eat. But ultimately the vast blankness of night or brightness of day are beyond my attention.

Fanned out before me are recondite texts on anxiety disorders, anoxia, pacemakers, postcardiotomy, anything that has to do with my unique history. It strikes me as ironic that I can concentrate on medicine that is tangential to my own condition in the privacy and quiet of the library, but am unable to tolerate the presence of others in the lecture hall. In spite of the close physical and intellectual proximity, medical school seems a long way off.

Beginning that week I meet with Dr. Gaensbauer, another strikingly shy psychiatrist. His voice is an apprehensive mumble and his manner always self-effacing. If I make the slightest utterance or hint at the will to speak while he is speaking, he automatically defers. Twice each week we meet in his small office in the brick psychiatry building and discuss the symptoms, my family's genetic history, fear of my pacemaker malfunctioning, the nature of being, my inability to view the blood scenes of surgery, and how I might one day learn to cope. I see a thin ray of hope penetrating the void; my life grows narrow in focus, laser-like out of necessity. I now understand that any aspect of my former life is not possible until I find out what has robbed my mind of its former discipline and integrity. So I leave behind all I once loved. I realize that I cannot become a doctor because I know too intimately the pain and terror of the patient; I identify instead of empathize. Hope, as I once knew it, is not possible until I heal myself.

During one of our visits I share with him my discovery that the Valium he has prescribed provides only limited relief, and sometimes no relief at all. However, I have found something that works flawlessly: Kentucky bourbon. One shot and I am terror-free for an hour; two shots and I feel I could endure torture sessions in an NVA prisoner-of-war camp and have a lovely time. Yet I know of the dangers of indulging in alcohol, and Gaensbauer agrees that the temporary cure would prove more damaging than the disease, so I should stay the hell away from it. He doesn't have to convince me; I want no part of it.

Late one night as I lie curled into the arm of a sofa reading a journal on the postsurgical effects of the heart-lung machine, I happen across an ailment called postcardiotomy syndrome. The list of symptoms includes loss of concentration, impaired memory, irritability, disorientation, altered perception, severe anxiety, and mild paranoia, all of which decrease with time and usually resolve themselves within six months of the surgery. The syndrome is partly a result of being on the heart-lung machine for too long, as I was, during which time the brain is starved of oxygen. The list of symptoms doesn't account for my flashbacks or feelings that I am separated from my surroundings, nevertheless I feel triumphant, believing I have solved a small part of the vast puzzle.

Later in the week while reading of neurological complications I discover a set of symptoms that specifically fits into a diagnosis called temporal lobe seizures. I consult Dr. Gaensbauer along with a professor of neurology at the medical school and they both agree to have me tested for minimal brain dysfunction and seizure activity. A battery of tests is given that test memory, motor skills, and concentration, and shows that mild insult to the brain has occurred. However, the damage sustained on the operating table is so mild and, they believe, temporary, that it couldn't possibly be the root of my problem.

So with Dr. Gaensbauer I delve into my past, sorting through parcels of pain and anger floating through the vast emptiness. The thoroughness of the inquiries is at first unsettling, but gradually my familial past is merged into my own study and together we arrive at the premise that the severe trauma and my own past have combined into a condition of both a physical and psychological nature. The symptoms of anxiety and depression are a result of a sad and traumatic life rooted in the blood.

Dr. Gaensbauer brings up the fact that for twenty years I haven't thoroughly grieved my mother's death, nor hardly thought of her at all, yet her memory is in my flesh. He asks me in various ways what I think about that as a theory, but my answer can only be expressed in tears.

The physical trauma, Dr. Gaensbauer emphasizes, is temporary and pales in comparison to the emotional. Physical injuries are mere flesh wounds; it is the psychological terror bred in my past that is most lethal. The catastrophic events that have directly threatened my life are what's causing the anxiety and depression. He says all this with a directness and confidence that both frightens and inspires.

"So the enemy has been identified," I say.

"We can see his silhouette."

But for the next few months the symptoms do not diminish to any appreciable degree, and some days they worsen. Late one afternoon while making a bold expedition to the supermarket a mysterious phenomenon occurs. While cautiously propelling a grocery cart down the aisle, an attack of panic comes furiously rushing back, and again I sense the familiar dislocation. For several minutes it is as though a rain-splattered windshield has come between myself and the surrounding aisles. The passing faces of shoppers melt into menacing grotesques, villainous in aspect, the environment is tinged with hostility. I feel at last I am insane, I am forever lost in a world of illusions and delusions. I quickly abandon my grocery cart, make my way through the door and scramble to the security of my car. By the time I arrive home I am convinced this is some form of schizophrenia* that is

---

*Schizophrenia includes a group of disorders which produce recurrent or chronic psychoses (inability to recognize "reality") characterized by bizarre, idiosyncratic thinking and thought disorganization, accompanied by hallucinations and delusions. It is now thought by modern psychiatrists that the roots of schizophrenia probably lie within the realm of organic brain diseases. The terrifying disorder is treatable, but unfortunately as of yet incurable.

producing this world of distorted faces and smudged reality. Not until my next session with Dr. Gaensbauer do I leave my apartment.

When we meet three days later he is skeptical. I give him a thorough account of the symptoms, but he only nods sympathetically and reiterates his belief that I'm now wandering off track. The discussion grows into a gentle argument with both of us equally certain of our positions, and Dr. Gaensbauer finally capitulates. With a kind of smug composure he suggests that I enter a transitional care program at the University Hospital for schizophrenic patients who have recently been released from the psychiatric ward. He rotates about in his swivel chair, makes a quick phone call, and after hanging up, he glibly parts his hands as if to say, done.

One morning a few days later I head for the transitional care department with my head down, eyes on the gray slabs of sidewalk, averting gazes and attention. And what happens through the course of the next two weeks I never share with Richard nor anyone in the family simply because I am too ashamed. What I see upon my arrival I am utterly unprepared for. Shaking and frightened and meek, I am shown a seat by the director in the midst of a group of men and women whose suffering is so flagrantly pronounced that I instantly identify with them, yet suspect that we indeed suffer at the hands of different illnesses. Their faces are expressionless, what psychiatrists call a flat affect. But what is most striking and haunting is their consistent response to sights and sounds that simply are not there. Again I think of R. D. Laing's theory concerning the reality of schizophrenics—that these withdrawn and frightened human beings are quite possibly the most sensitive of us all, that their private world is perhaps as real or unreal as the madness of the world we all endure. The only real thing I share with these people is their terror; yet theirs is constant and, as far as the medical world is concerned, permanent. There is no escape from the schizophrenic's house of specters.

At times I feel our terror is quite mutual. In the afternoons we are led out to the grassy courtyard by the director where we kick a large red ball between ourselves or wander about the grounds at the prompting of imaginary voices and faces. These days are fixed in the fabric of memory in a light that is a little overexposed for madness, the lush spears of bluegrass almost silver, the sky yellow-white with a more intense sunlight. The strange brightness suggests the madness of nature, its terrifying beauty, that terror is the essence of beauty.

One afternoon in the courtyard of the psychiatry building I am struck by a scene that will remain indelibly painted in my mind's eye. As I kick the large red ball with another patient I see two medical students rushing toward us down the sidewalk. About their necks hang stethoscopes, under their arms are manila folders of X rays. Then as they come closer I recognize one of the guys as a former classmate of mine. Our eyes meet, their conversation stalls, his animated expression goes flaccid. Eyes upon eyes. No words are spoken as they drift by, but the communication is clear: Poor Pensack, they fucked him up good—he would have been a good doctor, now look at him. He's ruined. I turn away once they've passed, look down at the red kickball in the grass, the spring foliage, then gaze at the mad and simple activities of my new friends.

After two weeks of this life Dr. Gaensbauer's treatment has achieved its desired effect. The fact that I can appreciate all my symptoms, including the visual and auditory disturbances, as insane distinguishes me from the true schizophrenic. The world of the schizophrenic is recognized by them as reality, whereas my world I recognize as a distortion of reality. I return to regular psychotherapy sessions, and days and evenings in the library. One afternoon while rummaging through the card catalogue I come across a book entitled *Fears and Phobias* by Isaac M. Marks. I settle into the familiar posture of the sofa with its lumpy fill and compressed springs then attack the text with a new vigor and awareness. A section of the book concerning agoraphobia describes my fear of leaving the apartment and going to loud or crowded places. It was described in ancient times and in Greek means literally "fear of the marketplace." I'm struck by the accuracy, that it is all here—my fear of faces in the supermarket, the suffocation of decorum, the illusions of hostile, menacing faces. My symptoms fall under different syndromes as I read on, but all come under the umbrella of fears and phobias induced by trauma. Case studies are offered, even by Burton who describes Hippocrates as a man who "loves darkness as life, and cannot endure light or to sit in lightsome places. . . . He dare not come in company, for fear he should be misused, disgraced, overshoot himself in gesture or speeches, or be sick; he thinks every man observes him." Exactly.

As I read I imagine Hippocrates found it impossible to eat or drink in front of others, being unable to swallow for fear of appearing ridiculous, and he too was afraid to be seen for fear of appearing awkward. But toward the end of the book Marks points out that talk psychotherapy only improves the patients' insight into their own behavior, but never cures, or extinguishes, their symptoms. He goes on to suggest a treatment that involves desensitization therapy accompanied by medication that helps block panic. The drugs are medical compounds known as tricyclic antidepressants. For reasons that at the time are not entirely understood, they seem to lessen the severity of panic, and have recently been approved by the FDA. Desensitization therapy was first explored by Dr. Joseph Wolpe at his clinic in Philadelphia in 1958, and consists of visualizing anxiety-provoking scenarios while either hypnotized or very relaxed. Eventually the patient is taught to actualize the state of calm in the real world—that is, in the marketplace.

So with the help of Dr. Gaensbauer, along with another therapist who specializes in desensitization therapy, and a biofeedback machine, I slowly become adept at controlling my own physiology (my blood pressure, heart rate, sweating response, etc.) while wired to the maze of apparatus. If I can incorporate a degree of this learned serenity into fearful situations, then I may be able to cancel out the anxiety, we agree. And this is precisely what I work toward for the next few months. Though I never conquer the symptoms entirely, I manage to leave the house by an effort of concentration, reminding myself that the menacing forces of nature and society are merely smoke and mirrors, a trick my mind plays on itself. These images do not represent reality, they cannot hurt me. From time to time I even make symbolic expeditions by car.

One summery and hot afternoon I leave for Boulder to walk around the campus with the expectation that the combination of a familiar setting and the relaxed summer school crowd will provide a therapeutic mix. And it does. A hot wind pours through campus, swaying the elms and cottonwoods, students sally along the sidewalks, relaxed and at ease in their bell-bottoms and Birkenstocks. I feel hints of nostalgia, a refreshing emotion. After an hour of aimless wandering I walk to the student union and buy a large cup of iced tea then take a seat in the cafeteria. As the panic shows itself, to calm myself I concentrate on the beads of sweat collecting against the waxed cup. A few tense minutes pass and the fear vanishes. Then I gaze about and see someone who seems vaguely familiar approaching down the hallway. He's a young black student whom I'm certain I know; the familiarity grows downright eerie as he approaches. I watch him order from the grill, then walk with his tray to a table with a slender book wedged in his armpit. As he comes closer I see his face is puffy, and it strikes me all at once who this guy is. In a moment of daring, I walk up to his table and address him as he raises a ham and cheese sandwich to his mouth.

"Excuse me, but is your name Steve?"

"Sure is."

"I know you from a few years back. You were a patient of Dr. Starzl's at the University Hospital."

"How'd you know that?"

"I dialyzed you when you were in pretty bad shape. I hate to say this, but I thought you were dead."

He smiles and looks me up and down.

"I received a second kidney from my brother back in October of 1973."

"Well, it's good to see you're doing all right." I fidget and prepare to turn and leave.

"So do you still work at the hospital?" he asks.

"No. I just dropped out of medical school. I've had some health problems of my own."

"Really?" He appears astonished. "I've applied for medical school in the fall."

"Wonderful, that's really great," I say, working up an appropriate smile. "Well, I plan to join you . . . you know, sometime soon."

We exchange nods and say goodbye.

Back in Denver I tell Dr. Gaensbauer that I need out of the city, away from the school, away from medicine. I tell him I've seen an ad in the *Denver Post* about a new juvenile child care facility near Steamboat Springs on Rabbit Ears Pass where I could help counsel troubled adolescents. I tell him how I imagine the setting as being quiet, tranquil, pristine. He says it may help, but that it would be best if we kept meeting once a week, and I agree.

So that afternoon I type up a résumé, send it off in the mail, and a week later I'm called up to Steamboat Springs for an interview. I'm nervous, a bit shaky, but I treat the interview as a session with Dr. Gaensbauer. I tell the panel of staff about my medical history, how I've been shaken from recent events, and how I could be of service to myself and these kids. Before leaving I'm offered the job and shown my new quarters. Off on an arm of the lake is a quaint but tattered log cabin with a small wooden porch sloping down toward the water's edge.

That evening I drive back to Denver and the following week I make the move to this remote camp called Leichen, which is run by an order of Episcopal monks. Here in an atmosphere distilled above nine thousand feet on the shore of a mountain lake I begin to feel my heart and mind healing. The days quickly fall into a soothing routine of mornings and afternoons spent by myself or with a friend, and the evenings with kids that have clearly taken to me. Together we set up a boxing bag and spar against each other, learn the delicate technique of a speed bag, the science of what on the surface appears to be barbaric. Monks silently wander about the grounds, heads bowed, hands clasped behind their woolen medieval robes. At night a friend on the staff, Gene Mahoney, and I sit on the porch of my cabin and quietly watch the harvest moon arc across the night sky over the ripening aspen leaves. This is my first new friendship since the surgery. From the beginning we speak to one another in hushed voices, with Bob Dylan songs oozing through the warped wooden door of my cabin. Spread out before us is the lake with an image of the moon tracing a silver path across the glassy surface, and the gentle lapping of waves. In the early-morning hours Gene and I will take a rowboat out on the lake with our fishing rods, and spend the quiet hours in coves teasing brookies with flies. During the late fall the waters cool, the trout slow and I go out by myself and let the boat glide through the water, trailing an arm in the cool surface. Then through the winter months the camp is submerged in snow, the dense whiteness muffling all sound, stilling all movement.

At first none of the children know of my heart condition, though the word eventually gets around. When I box and the sweaty shirt clings to my abdomen, the shape of the pacemaker can be made out. The kids are stunned when it is explained to them what the device does and that it keeps me alive. They are awed, amazed that I would risk my life boxing with them, and I in return am grateful for their appreciation. But at the end of the year the school runs into difficult financial times and it is announced that it will close in June. So I make the move back to Denver, uncertain about what I should do next. Although I'm improving emotionally, I know I'm not yet ready to return to school.

It's been a year and a half since the surgery and already I've had episodes of atrial fibrillation similar to, though not as severe as, the attack that knocked me out on the football field four years ago. Whenever it occurs, I concentrate on relaxing, mentally going to another place and time while telling myself this won't kill me. In June of 1977, Richard underwent the same septal myotomy and myectomy performed by Dr. Morrow as well. He too had suffered from episodes of fainting, light-headedness and dangerous arrhythmias, which had been increasing in severity and frequency. The surgery itself did not result in the need for a pacemaker, though the dangerous arrhythmias still persist.

Back in Denver the symptoms of fear, panic and unreality continue to seep through the veil of everyday life, though I now manage them better. I know the symptoms of my heart condition and shattered psyche aren't going to just go away. Also, the pacemaker imbedded in my belly paces my abdominal muscles

at the rate of seventy beats per minute whenever my own conduction system fails. It goes without saying that it requires a
certain measure of concentration simply to achieve sleep on quiet
summer evenings.

But at least the pacemaker problem is solvable. Again I return
to the library where I learn the mechanics of pacing systems and
discover it's quite an involved science, one that is improving almost yearly. Early on in my reading I learn that what I've got
prompting my heart to beat is a dinosaur, one of the more primitive models available; what I want is something that at the very
least won't test my concentration.

Late in the month I leave for the NIH armed with a folder of
mimeographed articles on pacemaker systems which I present to
the cardiology staff. What I want, I tell them, is a bipolar, not a
unipolar pacemaker, which impresses them immensely (the
bipolar will eliminate the twitching of my abdominal muscles).
This, they assure me, is not a problem, and later in the week I am
scheduled in for surgery to have such a device implanted. For
those three days before the surgery the question of whether or
not I can stand the sight of blood—my own blood—comes to
mind. I want to test myself, quantify my progress through the
past eighteen months. Before returning to my third year of medical school, the clinical year during which such bloody scenes are
commonplace, I'll need to view bloodletting with thorough
equanimity. What I'm afraid of is failure, of losing my head and
living with the certainty that becoming a doctor is no longer
possible. But when the day comes and I'm wheeled into the OR
suite I once again ask the attending surgeon if a mirror could be
placed so that I might observe the surgery. He's shocked. He
looks at me as though I belong in a circus or freak show, a maso-
chist worthy of medical attention. Before he answers I explain
that I was a medical student and plan on returning as soon as this
pacemaker is up and running, and that my interest is purely an

academic one. This puts him at ease. His kneaded temples relax, he shrugs his shoulders and says with mock indifference, "Suit yourself."

Soon the procedure is under way with a surgical nurse holding a rectangular mirror over the surgeon's gloved hands. I practice my relaxation techniques as the local anesthetic is administered through multiple-needle injections, my mind calmly telling itself that I am safe despite the fact that my life is being tinkered with before my very eyes. I measure my pulse in my ears, unclench my hands, and free the moistened fingers so that they might radiate heat. In the wedge of mirror the skin is parted along the seam of the old scar and the ruby flesh revealed. All I feel is a shadow of pressure, all I see is a phantom wound. My previous inability to witness such scenes when inflicted on others, I assume, has been vanquished. I am now both identifying and empathizing because I know it is me beneath the knife in the mirror, my own flesh and blood. A crisis has been resolved. After a few graceful lacerations into the valley of the wound the titanium casing of the pacemaker is revealed and I see for the first time the machine that has become a part of me.

24

Days later I am on the New Jersey shore with my old friends
John and Ted Ritota. They introduce me to a twenty-one-year-
old girl in a turquoise bikini, a Jewish girl by the name of Abbe
Singer. Together we exchange witticisms; a wonderful flirtatious
banter develops. She challenges my caustic sense of humor with a
dry wit.

We boys are all shirtless, the sun striking our reddened white
skin. From my abdomen the four-day-old wound is weeping between the sutures and the precise shape of the new pacemaker is
plainly visible. As the conversation continues from the ludicrous
to the absurd, Abbe and I exchange a staccato of outrageous and
undignified one-liners that go back and forth like bursts of ma-
chine-gun fire. She puzzles me. Here is a beautiful, olive-skinned
Semitic girl in a brilliant turquoise bikini who doesn't appear
to notice my new wound. Either she doesn't notice or she
doesn't care. But it is grotesquely prominent and nobody's that
oblivious.

Through the day we drink beer, walk along the beach of
grainy white sand and talk with a wonderful languid ease that I
haven't experienced for many years. I feel as though I am once
again at home in the world. As the sun swings over the ocean and
into the trees we all head to Max's Hotdogs and eat together on
picnic tables before yellow fluorescent lights and the screen door.
The humid evening carries the sounds and smells of midsum-

mer. When we finish eating everyone announces they've got to be going, so I offer to drive Abbe home. With my father's black Targa we ease through the cool summer evening air. When we arrive I ask for her phone number and tell her I'd like to get together before flying back to Colorado. "Certainly," she says. There is no kiss, no hug; only the gentle report of the door, and her small brown hand waving goodbye as she glides up the sidewalk to her apartment.

Three days later I call the number she scrawled on the back of an envelope and with a solid confidence I ask her to dinner at a Japanese steakhouse, followed by a party with John Ritota and our friends. Without a trace of restraint in her voice she accepts and we agree that I'll pick her up at five o'clock. At dinner small ceramic cups of saki are passed around, the warm colorless wine subduing any nervousness before Abbe who is stunning in her pink dress. She is someone I need not be compelled to feel self-conscious around—tipsy or sober. Oversized bottles of Japanese beer are brought out with dinner by the small and gracious proprietor, and the evening launches into bawdy jokes and laughter. Then after dinner we leave for the party at the home of John Ritota's friend who, John explains, is involved in some vague business affairs. Our host is also extraordinarily wealthy with an elegant home. The tone of this background on our host enlivens the atmosphere, tainting it with the romantic spirit of a film noir.

As we drive there in our caravan of three cars the ruddy summer sun is setting in the trees, the evening heavy with anticipation. When we arrive we are greeted by men in silk suits and led through a palatial estate to the marble patio surrounding a swimming pool. I ask John what it is precisely that his friend does for a living and he replies in a secretive whisper, "He's a businessman." Abbe's and my eyes widen with this revelation.

Just inside the house stands a full wet bar complete with a bartender. As the evening passes the patio area fills with guests, the music grows loud, and everyone becomes giddy with drunkenness. Abbe and I mill about the crowd as a couple, her presence at my side consistent evidence of her affection. We talk together about our host who has the appeal of a Gatsby-like character, as he is seldom seen and virtually unknown by nearly everyone but John and Ted, yet he is generous to utter strangers. Eventually we see him standing with a lady guest in the imprecise shadows of a willow at the far end of the pool, a young man strangely removed and elusive by nature.

As the hour grows late the party builds a momentum all its own. Well after midnight suitcoats, pants and dresses are discarded and the pool inundated with marauding bodies and hysterical laughter. At some point amid the chaos of voices and flailing swimmers I ask Abbe if she'd care to leave, and she takes my hand and nods. Outside where the Targa sits invisible in the darkness, the night is alive with the racket of locusts and crickets. When we step into the car Abbe notes that it's 2:00 A.M. with suppressed alarm.

"You'll be getting to bed late tonight," she says.

"No later than you."

The car hums, almost catlike, as it speeds down the empty Garden State Parkway to Abbe's apartment that lies thirty exits away. An hour later the headlights of the Targa are swinging across the darkened suburban homes as we coast beneath the streetlights. I pull up, kill the engine immediately and offer to walk her to the door. As she turns and sleepily wobbles up the sidewalk I discreetly pull out my small green overnight case from behind the driver's seat, then meet Abbe beneath the electric porchlight at her front doorstep. There is a moment of awkward silence, then I take her into my arms and tell her I had a wonderful time.

"Me, too," she says, her voice weak with sleeplessness. Then her head collapses into my chest.

"How about if I call you again before I fly back to Colorado?"

"Sure." She yawns, her delicate mouth drawing in the cool night air. After a brief pause I bring my mouth to hers, cautious, then there is a long intimate kiss, which has the effect of momentarily waking us both. Then as our mouths part she notices that I have this overnight bag in my right hand. For a moment she looks puzzled, almost worried.

"What's that in your hand?" she asks.

"How do you expect me to brush my teeth in the morning?"

Morning light pours through the thick brocaded curtains, imbuing the room with a dark rich Lincoln green. The white lace of Abbe's nightgown brilliantly contrasts her tanned skin as she lies facedown in a maze of pillows. I sit up and wonder for a moment what it was that woke me after only a few hours of sleep. I estimate by the shallow angle of sunlight and the utter stillness of the neighborhood beyond the curtains that it is still early. Then I sense the general weariness. For the past several days I've felt sluggish, particularly when exercising. I delicately try to ease out of bed and make my way to the bathroom, feeling the steady pace of my heart in my ears. Then something occurs to me. I stand before the mirror observing the scars, running my fingertips over the toughened perforations. Since the day on the beach, my heart rate hasn't been above seventy beats per minute, the rate of the pacemaker. My heart's own conduction system is not working. I am now and forever dependent upon the pacemaker for every heartbeat. The suspicion is strong, druglike in its effect. "Well now," I say to the image in the mirror, then head back to the bed where Abbe is stirring in her sleep. As I crawl over her legs beneath the heap of bedding she awakens.

"Do all medical students get by on just a few hours' sleep?" Her voice is groggy.

"It was a way of life."

"What time is it?"

"Early. Six or seven."

To my surprise she sits up, erect and alert, and shakes her long dark hair. Her eyes are clear and well-rested.

"You know, I think something's wrong," I say, trying to hedge any note of alarm in my voice. Her forehead crimps with vague concern; she's now fully awake.

"What's that?"

"You know this thing in my abdomen," I say, holding a thumb and forefinger about the canister, "this thing that looks like I keep a travel clock under my skin? Well, I think it's the only thing keeping my heart going."

"Isn't that what it's supposed to do?"

"Yeah, but it used to kick in only when my own heart stopped keeping pace. Now it's on all the time."

"How do you know?"

"Because my heart rate won't go above seventy beats per minute, which is what the pacemaker is programmed at." I throw my hands up and try to smile. "I'm tired all the time now."

"Well, what should we do?"

I look at her for a moment without saying a word. I like the word "we."

"Could you give me a lift to the hospital?"

That afternoon the doctors confirm what I already suspected: I am in complete heart block. My own conduction system that was injured during the heart surgery nearly two years ago now no longer works at all. My life now depends on this little clock keeping my heart beating for the rest of my life. I try not to let the knowledge bother me at first by simply directing my thoughts elsewhere, such as in Abbe's direction. But I'm fatigued constantly, my heart unable to speed up when commanded to do so by aching muscles, and forgetting proves impossible. Meanwhile there is a love affair to be conducted.

For the next ten days Abbe and I are inseparable, and we fall deeply and, unbeknownst to us, irrevocably in love. Were it not for this curious young girl who appears not only unfazed by my scarred and disfigured body, but actually interested in the mechanics of my heart, I would no doubt be frightened out of my mind. But for the next ten days it is made clear to me that I am no longer alone in this world.

Yet as the day of my departure approaches, the old sense of worry and dread creeps into my mood. The ocean that days before looked so vigorous and rejuvenating now appears gray and exhausted under sunny skies. And my departure date finally arrives.

With her hair pulled up into a casual summer ponytail, Abbe comes speeding up the quiet suburban street in her yellow Volkswagen fastback and halts before my parents' home. She walks to the door where I meet her with my suitcases on either side of me. Without a word she kisses my cheek then her small hand grips a suitcase handle and she is hauling it down the sidewalk to the car. Within minutes we are on the freeway, zigzagging through traffic to Newark Airport.

Few words are exchanged, perhaps because it has been left unclear as to what the past ten days were—love or fun? When we do speak there are turgid pauses filled with the overwhelming rage of a Volkswagen engine being forced to its very limits. Then there is the airport, the control tower looming over the bands of concrete and jumbo jets squatting on the tarmac. She pulls the car up to the United concourse and leaves it idling while we each carry a suitcase to the ticket counter. The sounds of an airport surround us—overlapping P.A. systems, conveyer belts, the echo and hum. We say goodbye, maybe we'll see each other again, then kiss, and I am off again, soaring toward the Rockies.

The first order of business back in Denver is returning to the library and finding a more sophisticated pacing system that my particular condition would be improved by. If my heart won't pace itself, I'll find the very best machine that will do it for me. The first name I ever wrote down in conjunction with pacemakers was Dr. Benjamin Rosenberg, located at the Presbyterian Medical Center, the very hospital where my mother died in 1955, and Richard and I were born. My father has told me Rosenberg's father was our mother's physician. As I read I invest the name and place with a pithy meaning. I picture my mother mouthing the name, *Dr. Rosenberg.*

One afternoon I write a letter of introduction to him and explain my medical history and what it is I need. As I understand my problem, the S.A. node, the miraculous piece of tissue that initiates the electrical activity of the heart's upper chambers, still works just fine. The problem is that the impulse never gets through the A.V. node, which functions as a relay terminal, to the ventricles due to the injury incurred during my surgery. So what I need is a machine that will send the impulse initiated at the top of the heart to the lower chambers, thereby coordinating the electrical activity from top to bottom. At the time these dual-chambered pacing systems are the state-of-the-art, but are believed by Dr. Morrow at the NIH to be undependable. A week later I receive Dr. Rosenberg's reply. He concurs with my opinion concerning what I need, and states that the pacer I have in mind is in fact quite dependable, as he has been implanting them routinely for two years now. He encourages me to call and discuss my case further, and I do. Over the phone an appointment is arranged for October.

The news makes me ecstatic. I write Abbe to tell her that I'll be seeing her again soon, and she promptly writes back. An exchange of letters begins with the word "love" surrounded by expressions of infinity. Through the haze of the next few weeks stretches of depression and melancholy are broken by scented envelopes that lie among bills and other meaningless correspondence. Yet there is the heart that will not speed up nor slow down, coupled with the stubborn symptoms of profuse sweating, shaking and a fantastic fear of the everyday—all of this in the face of joy. For now this hopeful future lies impaled upon the present, withering but not dying.

So I make other plans that, for the time being, I disclose only to Dr. Gaensbauer. I decide that now is the time to get back into medical school, I need to become a solid citizen of this planet, one with a plan and a purpose. This madness isn't going to go away entirely anytime soon, so waiting around is little more than pounding dirt down a rathole. I've been out of school for two years now. I tell Dr. Gaensbauer I want to accomplish three other things while back east: heal my mind, get a new pacemaker, and fall in love with Abbe. Dr. Gaensbauer tells me in his quiet soothing tone that if I really think I'm ready, then it's time to talk with the dean.

The following afternoon I head to the administrative offices where the dean greets me with expansive happiness, a kind of rugged tenderness. He offers me a seat before his immense desk and I begin a narrative of the last two years, and of my new plans. An expression of visceral satisfaction, a serene grin, forms across his mouth and sets in his eyes as I speak. He sits quietly and patiently as if waiting for me to say the words, "It's time to consider returning." When I do, he lightly claps his hands together and says, "Congratulations, Bob." Of course, he tells me, I'll need to study for and pass the first part of the National Medical Boards, in order to begin my third year, the first clinical year, of medical school the following fall.

"I'll be heading to New Jersey for the pacemaker operation next month, so I'll need to study there," I tell him.

"I know the dean at Rutgers. Perhaps you could sit in on classes."

"That's in New Brunswick?" I ask.

"That's right."

"Perfect."

He reaches for his Rolodex, then the phone and speaks nostalgically with his old friend and finally hangs up.

"Well, there you go, Bob."

Two weeks later Abbe is waiting at the end of a crowded concourse, wearing a woolen coat and scarf. Her silver and turquoise earrings glitter through the waves of her hair. My heart quickens as I move toward her.

For the next few days we hole up in her apartment at night; by day I look for a place to live, sign up for classes, and meet with Dr. Rosenberg while Abbe is away at work. I still need isolation, a buffer between me and the world of arbitrary stimuli and accidents. For days Abbe and I sift through newspapers, make phone calls, ask about farmhouses buried in open space that might allow my mind to calm itself. But such places on the East Coast are far too expensive.

Then one day while speaking with the dean of the medical school he tells me of a college history professor who is planning to take a sabbatical for the year and needs a student to watch after his farmstead and horse. That afternoon I make an appointment to meet the professor and his wife at their home which lies just outside of Cranbury, New Jersey. As I coast up the driveway in Abbe's fastback, I see on a wrought-iron post a placard that declares the estate an historical landmark, and that reveals it was constructed in 1774. The house itself is built of ancient white shingles with tiny windows and doorways. Outside in the barnyard I see an old man with hoary silver hair and a handlebar mustache feeding his horse oats from a plastic bucket. When I step out of the car he hobbles over in his Wellington boots and introduces himself as the professor.

That afternoon he and his wife spend the day leading me through this house of ghosts and thick spiderwebs with its overpowering Gothic aura. Everything is antique, including this couple, with their eighteenth-century sensibilities and their enormous house honeycombed with little rooms and stunted ceilings. Toward the end of the tour they make it clear that they would appreciate it if I looked after their place for the year and I gladly accept.

Life has been jump-started: through the quiet fall days I study with renewed concentration in the midst of the countryside like a mad English gentleman. In the late afternoon I will spot Abbe's car from the office window wobbling up the wash gravel drive, and together we take walks, watch the dense orange sun silently decline into the forest of hickory and ash. During the day my head possesses the pleasant ache of having focused on a network of theories that explains the human organism; then the walks with Abbe make for a pleasant reprieve and provide the security necessary for all stable human beings to feel they are not alone. The relative isolation is something we agree we could get used to. On these walks I describe to Abbe the colors and landscapes of the Rockies, the Western Slope.

Yet against the background of pastoral benevolence and gentility, there is still a surgery to be endured. Dr. Rosenberg isn't the tender and warm man who authored his letter and spoke to me over the phone. When we have spoken of my case in person it has been in the hallway only, a rapid, pressured and incomplete conversation. Always there is somewhere else he has to be. He is tall and lanky, with a coarse, Marine-like crew cut, and very distinguished in appearance. His hands I notice are shaped like those of Dr. Starzl—long, thin, beautifully feminine. It is difficult not to be impressed by the man. During one of these brief and unsatisfying conversations I explain to him that I not only want this new high-performance pacemaker, but if it's possible I would like a smaller one and have it moved from my abdomen to my chest. I begin explaining to him that I'm twenty-eight, have a new girlfriend and am still self-conscious about my appearance when with her; then he interrupts me and hurriedly says, "Sure, sure. It's not a problem. We'll implant a smaller one in your left axilla" [armpit]. Then he says he has got to be off.

"About how large will this one be?" I ask.

From twenty feet down the hall he says over his shoulder: "About the size of a cigarette lighter."

Talking to the man is like talking to god; you never feel you have his attention.

A few days later I arrive at the hospital ready to go under the knife. For the first time, really, Dr. Rosenberg sits down with me and explains the pacemaker and the procedure. Everything will be done under a local anesthetic; the pacemaker lead will be fed from my armpit through the subclavian vein into the heart where it will attach itself to the inside of the right atrium. And after several shots of novocaine, this is precisely what is done.

For a few days I am laid up in bed with wounds in my armpit, chest, and abdomen. After a day or two I manage to work my way out of bed and walk down the hall, and immediately I feel my heart speed up and slow down as I move about at the bidding of this fancy new pacemaker. With this knowledge, nothing can suppress my mood, as I know I have temporarily outwitted my disease. While exercising on a treadmill later in the week, I watch with a sort of static glee as I witness the increasing of my heart rate on the EKG tape and the monitor weaves a vigorous path.

When I am finally discharged I settle back into my former routine at the farmhouse, my genteel life as a country squire. It is now possible for my heart to accelerate to one hundred twenty beats per minute with the lurch of adrenaline or the desire to run. Yet whenever I go into town to shop, I realize that all the prior symptoms of anxiety and feelings of unreality are still there. This worries me. I know without a doubt that medical school is absolutely not a possibility until there is some sort of resolution to this problem.

One afternoon I attend a lecture on death and dying at Rutgers Medical School. The keynote speaker is a psychiatrist from Philadelphia by the name of Dr. John Fryer, an overweight, flamboyant yet eloquent academic. He speaks specifically of Elisabeth Kübler-Ross's theory on the five stages of dying, the moral and cultural importance of dying with a measure of dignity and not allowing the terminally ill to suffer. When he speaks of the various stages, I recognize myself in the allegory of experiences—denial, anger, bargaining with god, depression, and finally acceptance—though technically I am not afflicted with a "terminal" illness. Through the lecture I am mesmerized, gripped with rapt immobility as he describes, seemingly, my life. After the lecture it takes a moment to conjure up the courage to approach Dr. Fryer. But as students file out of the auditorium I abruptly introduce myself and begin relaying my medical and psychiatric histories as if reciting a movie script. His character, it seems, demands of him that he be remarkably approachable. He is clearly attentive and empathetic in a way that allows me to feel comfortable asking him if he would consent to see me as a patient if it fits into his schedule, and he graciously says he would be happy to. As he speaks I fix my eyes on his blood-red lips, his mobile mouth. He talks quickly, dramatically, accompanying the spoken word with gestures, the fluid grace of a fat man.

So once a week through the winter and spring I drive an hour and twenty minutes to Philadelphia where Dr. Fryer lives in Germantown. Every Tuesday I mount the broad steps of his Victorian home and sit in the waiting area with its lush velvet upholstery sofa and towering nineteenth-century portraits. The immense house is home to several medical students, all of them disciples of Dr. Fryer. On the ground floor is a commons area and a vast communal kitchen from which ardent conversations on esoteric theories concerning the life of the mind pour forth. The atmosphere is very Bohemian, very academic.

Our discussions progress along the same lines of thought as those I had with Dr. Gaensbauer, as they probe into my medical and familial past, seeking to extinguish fear with understanding. And to a degree this works; Dr. Fryer is a brilliant psychiatrist. He is so singularly focused on my story as he sits in his rumpled tweed jacket, his purpled lips and utterly pale face compressed in an effort of concentration. The contrast of his face and lips coupled with the Victorian decor of his office give our meetings a vampire-like atmosphere.

I fill him in on the desensitization therapy I've been involved with, and share with him my secret suspicions as to whether or not I am schizophrenic or preschizophrenic. After a few meetings I ask him point-blank if he thinks I am, and he replies slowly and thoughtfully, "I don't believe so." The uncertainty remains exasperating.

In the midst of winter, without any significant relief from the episodes of panic, I tell Dr. Fryer that I think I need to see a psychopharmacologist, someone who specializes in the drug management of psychiatric illness, and he agrees that it might be helpful. So one day I make an appointment with such a psychiatrist in New York City, then call my father to see if he would care to come along—and to my surprise he does. Perhaps it's that he is divorced now and is clearly feeling depressed himself.

Only in New York City could such a practice thrive. The hallways are lined with wealthy and crazy New Yorkers who, after spending a few minutes describing their symptoms to the psychiatrist, are prescribed medication to lessen or eliminate them. When my name is called, my father is instructed by the staff to wait in the reception area among the population of neurotic and psychotic* patients, which makes him uneasy. The psychiatrist, Dr. Anton Sonnheim, is fond of two-thousand-dollar Armani suits and Porsche shades. It is very appropriate, I think to myself, that he dresses like a drug kingpin. But the most ostentatious aspect of this man is his hair, which he slicks back with Brylcream and has tied into a ponytail. Before I have even sat down he tells me that he doesn't believe in the efficacy of talk psychotherapy, and in fact doesn't offer it. What he does offer is medication, and lots of it, though of course he doesn't say this. The only history he is interested in is my drug use in college, which wasn't very extensive—just a little marijuana every now and then—and a careful description of my presenting symptoms. I begin telling him of my cardiac problems, that I didn't have these symptoms before my cardiac arrest, but he cuts me off short and guides the discussion back to the college days. Then well within the hour he acts as though he has heard enough and

*Neurosis is a mental condition common to nearly all human beings resulting from unconscious internal conflicts, causing emotional turmoil that can lead to maladaptive behavior. Neurotics are aware of their unhappiness and are able to observe what part they themselves play in perpetuating it. Psychosis is a mental condition whose hallmark is an inability to recognize reality from unreality. It is marked by hallucinations (sounds and sights that are perceived by the patient as real, though they don't exist), delusions (fixed, false beliefs), and paranoia. As an old psychiatry professor once lectured, "Neurotics build castles in the sky, psychotics live in those castles, and psychiatrists charge the rent."

calls my father in to give us both his final opinion of what is wrong with me and how he plans to correct it. When my father arrives at the doorway, he appears profoundly relieved to be out of the waiting area.

"Well, Bob and I have had a very productive discussion," Dr. Sonnheim begins, his voice and manner very pontifical. "I'm going to begin treatment by prescribing two drugs to alleviate the severe anxiety he is obviously suffering from."

My father asks what it is that could have caused these severe symptoms of anxiety. The tone of certainty in Sonnheim's voice, the expression of his arrogance, piques my father's interest.

"Marijuana use," he says, parting his hands as though the answer were obvious.

There is a harrowing silence, as this medical opinion feeds into my father's preconceived notions concerning the dangers of marijuana.

All I can do is smile.

When not at the farmhouse I'm either in class or at the Rutgers Medical School library. I've applied to take the boards in the spring, which leaves me three months to prepare. And though there is an intense sense of urgency, a compulsive need to study 'round the clock, from time to time I am drawn to the periodical section of the library and continue researching anxiety disorders. The urge to focus on the subject is at times irresistible, particularly whenever the symptoms have recently recurred. Though I have no formal training in psychiatry, I feel infinitely more qualified than Dr. Sonnheim to treat myself.

For the first time I find literature on the relationship between panic, phobias, and trauma, the last of which seems to me to be the obvious culprit—not smoking marijuana—though until now I haven't made the conscious connection. If at times I am psychotic, I am so as a result of the trauma of multiple surgeries and my cardiac arrest which I witnessed; I feel rather sure of this. Until now this has been merely a vague suspicion, another unconscious belief.

After opinions from various so-called experts as to my underlying mental illness, a formal battery of psychological tests is ordered by Dr. Fryer at a psychiatric clinic. A week later I receive the results which are unequivocal. The report states that the symptoms are a result of a series of life-threatening experiences that have produced a very appropriate and overwhelming fear of death. The accumulation of trauma, the grisly memories, are causing these symptoms of distorted reality, feelings of impending doom, panic, and pervasive anxiety. To attribute them to occasional marijuana use years ago is absurd. The report, I feel, saves me. I am acquitted if not cured.

So I sink myself further into the Rutgers Medical School library researching the life of the mind at the expense of studying for the boards, and one afternoon I come across a reference to an article written in the early sixties by a preeminent English psychiatrist by the name of Sir Martin Roth, M.D. I immediately look up the original article entitled "The Phobic Anxiety Depersonalization Syndrome," and what I read astounds the senses. The walls and floor drop away, noises dissolve as my eyes consume the symbols on the page. Dr. Roth describes through case examples people who have endured life-threatening catastrophic events typically beyond the realm of common human experience. These people include accident victims who have witnessed the horror in the eyes of dying friends or family and went on to live and talk about it; they include soldiers, prisoners of war, Holocaust survivors. In the case histories I recognize myself, as I have lived beyond the realm of *common human experience.* These are people who have an irrational fear of leaving the house (phobic anxiety), people who cannot concentrate, experience distortions of reality, who have flashbacks of their respective traumatic events and suffer disabling panic attacks. All are accompanied by episodes of depersonalization.* In some extreme cases these people have experienced visual *and* auditory hallucinations—and they definitely are not schizophrenic. At once I recognize myself as a composite of these people, my experience an allegory of theirs. Then, in the vacant halls of a large library, I hear myself sobbing. From time to time people pass by the metal bookshelves as I gaze down through bleary eyes at the article. Eventually I collect myself and begin a long letter on yellow legal paper to Dr. Roth that explains everything about me, including my relief at having discovered his article. When I've finished I take it directly to the post office then drive back to the farm where I find Abbe curled up beneath a comforter before a small fire in the ancient stone fireplace. With a kiss to her forehead I wake her. As she emerges from sleep I show her the article and explain the significance of the discovery. During moments of silence the crackling of small wild flames fills the room.

"So you've treated your first patient, Dr. Pensack?" Her voice is sleepy.

"At least I've diagnosed him," I say. "That's more than anyone else has been able to do."

The next time I see Dr. Fryer I triumphantly present a photocopy of the article, and once he has carefully read it from beginning to end he agrees that I've correctly diagnosed my ailment.

Two weeks later I receive Dr. Roth's reply in the mail and he suggests that I continue with desensitization therapy. He states

---

*Depersonalization is a mental state characterized by feelings of unreality and strangeness. It can include bizarre feelings of detachment from one's environment, termed *derealization.* It can produce the sensation of being out of one's body and viewing oneself. It is a type of dissociative disorder, all of which generally result from psychological trauma.

that depersonalization is eminently treatable, though for me the greatest benefit lies in the knowledge that I am not chronically out of my mind.

Meanwhile the National Medical Boards loom just three weeks away. Through the days of late winter and early spring I sequester myself in the country with the scope of medical science explained in excruciating detail before me. Candleflames mix with a dull green lamplight and together brighten the dining room table littered with textbooks and mock exams. Abbe visits from time to time after work to help me prepare. The burden of information appears overwhelming and I grow panicked with self-doubt. The attenuation of days creates the illusion that I am hopelessly behind. My mood is hitched to my performance on the tests that Abbe gives me every evening as she lies swaddled in an afghan on the sofa. The days blur into a haze of nameless mornings and evenings, and when the test date arrives it does so with a degree of surprise. I show up at the Rutgers campus late and anxious, my mind roaming through the material—the rote memorization, the abstract theory—and when I am handed the exam I experience the familiar disorienting panic. Not until several minutes into the exam do I calm myself and dismiss all imaginary threats.

After eight weeks I check the mailbox at the end of the lane daily and try as best I can to relax and spend time with Abbe. We keep to ourselves at the farmhouse or go out with our small clique of friends and come to be recognized as a couple. We are Bob and Abbe. Then in early July of 1978 the mailman arrives in a little white truck and I walk out to the box, tear open the envelope to discover I've passed. Moreover, there is a letter of congratulations from the dean at the University of Colorado Medical School. I am going to be a doctor. It's been two and a half years since I left, but I'm going to be a doctor. I slowly walk back to the house, watching the mailman's truck rolling over the shallow hills in the distance, and meet Abbe inside. "I am going to be a doctor," I tell her.

It is understood I am going back to Colorado alone, back to two busy years of medical school. But before leaving, I arrive early one morning at Abbe's apartment, nervous and shaking, and I have her pour me a whiskey. There is a bit of nervous rambling, aimless speech uttered which Abbe patiently endures, then I ask her if she would be inclined to be my wife, to be Abbe Pensack. As if by simple and natural muscular reflex, she replies, "Of course."

25

I awake in darkness at 4:00 A.M. every morning, then Denver General Hospital to make pre-rounds at 5:00 A.M. For the next two hours I visit with patients, learn their individual case histories and confer with fellow students as to what their treatment should involve. One of these students, I learn, is Steve, the kidney-transplant patient I had dialyzed six years ago on Dr. Starzl's ward. He looks remarkably healthy, which makes me wonder if I am the only one who knows the commonality we share. The knowledge makes me suspect that everyone, every friend and stranger must come equipped with some fantastic secret, some terrible story. Very few know of my own illness, after all, since I've always appeared healthy.

After the pre-rounds our small group of medical students wanders from room to room with the chief resident who pumps us for information on each patient. What would you do for this patient if . . . ? How do you know that they are . . . ? The interrogation is tense, fast-paced and hostile if you are not thoroughly prepared. The best way to deflect the attention of the chief resident is to know your material. After the rounds I head for the operating room for eight or nine hours where the real test begins. One of the first operations I scrub in on is an aortic valve replacement, a procedure during which I will observe the throbbing of a glistening human heart. The initial incision is made, the chest slowly and unmercifully parted as I consciously check my breathing, trying to quell the force of adrenaline in my blood. Jokes are made, a return of the old grim humor that provides nervous release. Anxious laughter. At once I recognize this as a mechanism nearly all surgeons utilize to unconsciously separate themselves from the patient; perhaps it is also an expression of their own secret fear of mutilation. In this respect I am put at ease because I see that in a very essential way I am no different from anyone else in this suite. With this certainty in mind, I concentrate on my meager task of holding the retractors, and later I will actually hold the human heart in a steady hand. As the procedure wears on I sense a rich pride swelling up in me like a flame: I am doing what I was intended to do. I am once again becoming a doctor.

The pace of the schedule is ruthless. When on call we work for thirty-six hours straight then are off for eight. All of us live with a terrible longing to return home and submerge our aching minds in sleep, but that simply would not do. So we work as we never have before. But a few realities are made clear to me: there are certain fields of medicine that this heart will not tolerate. With fatigue comes chest pain, and from time to time, arrhythmia. If I am seeing a patient at the time or am with a group of people, I quietly close my eyes and search with my hands for a place to sit. As I feel the arrhythmia subside, the terror remains in my heart like dross, leaving its indelible stain. I meekly approach the chief resident, and by my pallor he asks with faint alarm what's wrong. Together we step aside and I speak candidly about my weary heart and the deadly side effects of sleep deprivation. Without much explanation the esprit de corps is suspended and I am ordered home to rest. So I go, weak, terrified and frustrated out of my mind. There is an unspoken code among medical students, one with the backbone of fortitude. In a fundamental way I feel separated by this invisible illness. My only consolation is the suspicion that Steve and others like us are in this together.

Nearly every day I talk with Abbe on the phone in New Jersey or write about mundane details of my day or imaginary scenarios of life after the ceremony this fall. At times I wonder if she understands what she's getting into with this marriage, because I know whoever chooses to love me will suffer at my side for the rest of our lives together. I am twenty-nine and she is twenty-two. I know that my future holds more corrective surgery, possibly even a heart transplant, events that could shatter any marriage. Moreover, I am in for an early death. I feel guilt over allowing her affections to go unchecked, but at the same time it is clear that she loves me in spite of my genetics. I remind her constantly how complicated the future could be, and she only looks forward to it with relish. The prospect of having children, however, is terrifying. We move around the subject in phone calls and letters delicately so as to keep the hope alive, yet with the reality I live with vaguely in mind.

Through the semester the arrhythmias grow more frequent and severe as the schedule intensifies. What I suspect is that this pacemaker is partly responsible for what is called reentry atrial tachycardia. After considerable research I suggest to Dr. Rosenberg in a letter that a more sophisticated pacemaker is needed to correct the problem, then he responds by saying I'm on to something, and invites me back to the hospital when medical school breaks for the summer.

So for the next six months my heart attempts to tolerate an assault of sheer wakeful hours. From time to time the weary muscle seems to grow confused as though from fatigue, and the arrhythmia often patters away deep within my chest, producing a tense ache and dizziness. I remain calm by talking myself through the invisible crisis, whispering with my eyes closed that everything is going to be all right, that the heart will soothe itself momentarily. And it always does.

In the meantime wedding plans are made for the fall at a country club. The exchange of letters between Abbe and me is frantic with bursts of apprehension, love, doubt and an intense hopefulness. I am going to need this pacemaker operation, I write her, before the wedding, so that we might start our lives with something new, something better than the past has offered us. She writes me back that the operation couldn't be more symbolically appropriate. A new ticker, a new watch to keep time by. Then the school year unmercifully comes to a close and I am on the first plane east and again flying toward Abbe.

A month before the wedding I am admitted into the hospital to have the newest pacemaker implanted, wholly expecting to be out in three days. The surgery itself proceeds without complication, and again I watch the operation as though for my own academic interest. I feel that witnessing the trauma inflicted upon my body will toughen the mind; what does not kill us only serves to make us stronger. That afternoon I am lying awake in bed with my fresh incision exposed as Abbe and my family visit, their voices floating all about me. I have the quiet satisfaction of a wounded soldier surrounded by friends and loved ones, safely removed from the front lines. And with me is my bride and my brother, who will be my best man. A new pacemaker, a fiancée, another year of medical school out of the way. I am on the mend. Richard and Linda have brought their infant son, Adam, along with them; they are a picture of a young Jewish family with their observance of tradition and the kosher home they now keep in New Jersey.

Then two days later, however, I am once again in an arrhythmia called atrial flutter. The Friday before Labor Day weekend, Dr. Rosenberg comes into the room to reprogram the new pacemaker before meeting his family in the Vineyard. As usual, he is in a terrific hurry. He has me undo my shirt and lie back as he produces the electromagnetic programmer from its box, and gives it a cursory inspection before sighing in general resignation and approaching my bed with it in his hands. Just beyond the blue curtain I can hear my father entering the room. He asks a nurse if I am here and she tells him in lay terms that Dr. Rosenberg is about to reprogram my pacemaker so that it will abolish the atrial flutter. The procedure is called atrial burst pacing and was done in the operating suite prior to the advent of this pacemaker. Rosenberg lowers the device over my chest and begins turning the dials in a seemingly random fashion. For a moment he grows impatient with the machine that isn't behaving predictably at his command. Then as he continues to work, I feel the effects of magnetism on my pacemaker. I stare at Rosenberg's thick crew cut as he mutters sharp authoritative curses, and the pace of my heart warbles to the wildly varying pitch of the programmer. Then, with terrifying suddenness, I feel my heart die in my chest and sense the old familiar fading of consciousness.

"My heart's stopping, it's stopping!" I hear myself shout.

Then all vision dims to blackness and there are only sounds of a frantic doctor and two nurses darting about the room. I hear Rosenberg shouting for the programmer manual, his voice threatening and rattled. I feel that immutable primordial stuff that binds body to consciousness slowly unravel and I begin drifting to that familiar and ubiquitous sea of calm. Before losing consciousness entirely, a singular thought passes through the emptied contents of my mind like a shaft of light: *Nothing is so easy as dying.*

Then there is the world before me. Dr. Rosenberg's grim and haggard face forcing a smile upon itself, my father's baffled and terrified voice from beyond the curtain, brightness and random tactile sensation. After a puzzling moment I feel the stream of tears on my face pouring onto my chest. Then the memory of fading consciousness, the dying of light, occurs to me in a tremor of panic. As I shiver with fear I gaze down at the floor where a pile of EKG tape has again documented the arrest of my heart.

"I was in asystole,* wasn't I?" I say, my voice clotted with tears.

"You were, but there's nothing to worry about now. You're all right. Everything's okay, Bob," Rosenberg says, forcing a smile.

Then there is my father's voice from behind the curtain. "Everything's all right, Bob. Dr. Rosenberg just had a little trouble with the programmer." His voice is strangely removed, full of contrived and formal reassurance. "But everything's fine now, son."

"Dad, they turned my heart off in here." My voice is terrified and angry. "Then they turned it back on. That's not all right."

The tenuous thread that connects spirit to body has shown itself for all its capricious and inconsequential purpose. The body has shown itself to be an electric organism that can be turned on and off.

In the aftermath of this terror, I fashion a theory that is still more unsettling, and I fear, correct. What many people who have experienced out-of-body sensations have touted as religious experiences are merely a form of depersonalization called *doubling*. The sense of floating over the room while your body is being revived as though your "spirit" has slipped from its physical cage below is well documented, and I can vouch for its occurrence. It is so well documented that I suppose it's quite universal, that is, everyone must experience some form of the sensation when at the brink of death. Though it may seem to be a glorious encounter with god, and widely interpreted as such, it is more likely a combination of the human's psychic defense

*No heartbeat, or arrest of the heart.

mechanisms, that is, a form of psychological denial. The emotional illusion is created that one is observing *somebody else.* The denial of one's death is a defense mechanism that protects us from the absolute terror inherent in the last moments of life. In addition, there is a biological explanation: when the brain is deprived of adequate oxygen, its function deteriorates, and this can be manifested through what appears to the dying organism as distortions of the environment. Ironic, I think, that we consider ourselves immortal right up to the very end, on the brink of death. Such is the theory of an entrenched agnostic and reluctant heretic.

26

Days before the wedding I am discharged from the hospital. Out of the hospital and down the aisle. The poignancy of the circumstances couldn't be more sharply demonstrated. Life is a naturally absurd phenomenon. In this light, death can hardly be viewed as a threat, I tell myself. There is no time to feel frightened, only to feel guilty; Abbe is marrying damaged goods, a man with a treacherous future laid out before him like a mined road.

The day before the ceremony, Abbe's mother speaks with her about the reservations she once had about her marrying a man with a chronic heart ailment. It is a repeat of all the reservations I have expressed to her but ends with a blanket endorsement of our love.

The families arrive on both sides from across the continent, including my cousin, Jessica, whose diabetes has slowly robbed her of sight. We spend our evenings talking of our mutual hospital experiences, what it means to suspect what you will one day die of. I tell her about my second cardiac arrest and Abbe's fears that I wouldn't get out of the hospital in time for the wedding, and the surreal bloody-red tincture that has tainted the ceremony. She listens without a word because she knows precisely about what I'm speaking. Toward the end of the conversation she commends me for keeping my head.

On the afternoon of our wedding, the sky is dull with high clouds, the autumn foliage sodden on the grounds of the country club. But as the day accomplishes itself, the sun leaks through in strands of light and gradually the weather breaks and moves over the sea.

Before walking down the aisle I walk into the clubhouse bar and ask the bartender for a double shot of bourbon. I don't have any money on me, I tell him, but I'm about to become a married man. And so he pours one for each of us and we toast to the brevity of life. After clapping the decanter down upon the mahogany bar, I abruptly turn to the door where the music has begun. A strange brightness fills the rectangular doorway, made so perhaps by the rush of alcohol through my veins, calming my naked anxiety. As I approach the door the wedding march commences and I am immediately propelled down the aisle beneath the *chupa* where Richard and I stand with the Rabbi, surrounded by white irises. Then Abbe appears at the far end of the aisle and we are married. A glass is carefully wrapped by Rabbi Cohen in a silk napkin, placed under my leather heel and crushed, a Jewish ritual to disperse the evil spirits. As the delicate figure of blown glass is ground into cusps I gaze over to Jessica, her weary eyes distorted behind thickened glasses, straining to witness the superstitious ceremony.

The following year I am possessed by a new security. I do not have to live this life alone as I am bonded to this woman through a covenant with a faceless god. We set up a house in Denver together which allows me to concentrate as I never have before on this medical career. When I arrive home late at night the house will be filled with the warm moist fragrance of leeks as the stew sits over a low flame in a pressure cooker on the stove. Quiet conversations fill our dining room beneath the soft light of the chandelier as we both lift the hot broth in spoonfuls, each of us thoroughly exhausted. Abbe works in the daytime as a travel agent then comes home to domesticate an empty house. The days become an exhausting and fulfilling routine of work and sleep. Then the following spring I graduate, and once again the family is brought together. After seven years of work and madness, after seven years of what ordinarily takes four, I become an M.D. at age thirty-one. The familiar faces of my past fill the audience: Jessica, my mother and father, Uncle Irwin and Aunt Judy, Abbe's parents, my grandmother Pensack. We file past the dean of students and are each handed a diploma, then after the regular ceremony I am presented with the Robert I. Slater Award as the student who has most demonstrated unusual dedication to medicine. My back is slapped, my eyes glisten as I mount the dais to accept the award. The reason I was chosen is not announced; as it has always been the family disease, it shall also remain a family secret.

I want to know it all, master the science of the human body, become intimate with its secret workings. As an intern I take rotations in general surgery, internal medicine, pediatrics, emergency room medicine, pathology and orthopedic surgery. Despite the fatigue and complications I experienced in medical school, I want to become a physician in the ancient sense of the word, one who is skilled in the art of healing, a *fisicien*. But every third or fourth night I am on call, working through thirty-six-hour stretches which are broken by nine-hour flashes of sleep. This brings on arrhythmias, usually in the form of atrial fibrillation. Late in the night I will doze in the call room for but a few minutes only to be awakened by the head nurse who will tell me I am needed in the coronary care unit. On a few of these occasions I am told a patient is experiencing life-threatening arrhythmia, while deep in my own chest I feel the sickening flutter of the same. In such cases I have a terrific expertise because I know quite specifically what treatment and drug therapy is required. When I describe the symptoms the patients are feeling, their eyes awaken with the intimate suspicion of shared knowledge, and I can see at once they are put at ease. I become skilled at this art of healing.

But with the episodes of fibrillation it is imperative that I take one or two days off until my heart converts to its regular rhythm with the help of medication. Prior to my internship, this occurred only once or twice a year, but now these episodes have gradually intensified in frequency and severity.

I learn to push on when feeling a little dizzy and complete the shift. After thirty-six hours I feel euphoric, manic, and become grandiose in gesture and thought. I become Superman. On Monday mornings I will awaken at 6:00 A.M. and not return home until 6:00 P.M. on Tuesday. At this point I will bring Abbe along with my fellow interns in a heightened spirit of invulnerability as we head out to a bar with the knowledge we are too numb for sleep. After an hour of buoyant frolicking, Abbe and I will move through the warm langourous residential streets beneath the moonlit shade trees and drift off to sleep in the grave darkness, our limbs entwined. Then comes the shrill cry of the alarm clock, and the cycle repeats itself.

During this time in a physician's training there is the pressure to specialize. Yet I wonder precisely what field of medicine this heart will be capable of withstanding. For some time now I have looked to psychiatry as the practical choice; psychological suffering is something I am acutely attuned to, and I find it intellectually fascinating. The interest is of course born of my history. The most intriguing aspect of the science is the study of brain function and its biological roots, and as a physician-psychiatrist one looks at human behavior not only from an emotional standpoint, but a biological one as well. This is the brave new world of modern medicine, this is the frontier.

However, choosing psychiatry as a specialty of medicine is viewed by many physicians as turning your back on all the training pertaining strictly to physical ailments that you have absorbed through the years. Real medicine involves blood and guts, sewing wounds, wearing a lab coat. Therefore psychiatrists abandon the physical and intellectual challenges presented by real medicine. All of this is of course absurd, but such opinions exist. Perhaps that is why I balk at making any hard-and-fast decision for several years concerning a specialty. I become a general practitioner and an emergency room physician who will see a lot of inner-city trauma by default.

There are times like these: at 3:00 A.M. I am awakened in the emergency room at St. Lukes Hospital in Denver and told by a nurse that a gunshot wound to the head just rolled in. I step out of the serene darkness of the call room to the panic and fluorescent lights of the ER where I am directed to a young black man with a dark brook of blood oozing down the side of his head. He is wide-awake, reeks of bourbon, knows what's going on, knows what has happened, but for some reason cannot verbalize it. His pupils are dilated though his vital signs are all stable. After getting IV lines into him, I order an X ray taken of his head which shows a .38 caliber bullet lodged in his right maxillary sinus, the space above the upper right jaw. When I take a second look at him I see the bullet has actually entered at the left side of his head just below the temple and impacted in the right. I call in the surgeons and he is promptly taken to the OR. When I return to the darkness of the call room at 5:00 A.M. I feel the nausea produced by the awkward flutter of my heart and lie down, listening to the sick thrusts in my ears. Before the day breaks I am awakened again, this time for a car accident. For three years I work in this setting while my heart threatens to strike me dead through the sleepless hours.

During my internship, I had come across a cardiologist by the name of Dr. Michael Sarché, a heart doctor with the uncanny combination of instinct and intelligence, compassion and compulsion. What separates him from other cardiologists I've met is his ability to listen to his patients' histories and to learn from them. By this time I feel I have been exposed to the greatest minds in medical science and most of them share one great fault which limits their ability. Their narcissism dictates that it is beneath them to listen to patients. Dr. Sarché is humble, even self-effacing; and he is also driven. Because of the intense professional interest I witness him take in his patients I place myself under his care. In my opinion he is as intelligent and knowledgeable as any cardiologist at the NIH.

One of his first prescriptions is a new experimental drug called amiodarone, an anti-arrhythmic with potentially severe side effects, including irreversible lung disease, thyroid disease, as well as bluish discoloration of the skin and photosensitivity. But the side effects of the drug pale in comparison to the symptoms of weakness and dizziness caused by atrial fibrillation. Within a few weeks the atrial fibrillation has ceased and I feel stronger than I have in ten years; suddenly I feel I can be any kind of doctor I want, the world unfurls. Before heading to the hospital, just as the day breaks, I will jog a few miles against doctors' advice, savoring the ache of actual muscle fatigue.

The following year I take more training in family practice in Cheyenne, Wyoming, where I work with another physician doing much of the obstetrical work. Again, every fourth night I am on call, nights that I effectively go without sleep, yet my heart tolerates the deprivation quite well at first. On the weekends I drive back to Denver, a two-hour drive south, to be with Abbe, then Sunday evening I head north again to deliver babies through the night. An extraordinary job, to be present during the first hours, the premiere of a life. The procedure becomes rote with the palpable force of miracle always there.

But as the days accumulate the symptoms return like faint ghosts in spite of the amiodarone. Early one morning after delivering my third baby, I feel an intense episode of atrial fibrillation shudder through my chest, and at that moment, as I lay myself down, sick and weary, I decide that it is time to move back to Denver and become a psychiatrist. In a sense I feel that is what I was meant to do anyway and what I always intended to be. The next morning I walk into the chairman's office, hand him my resignation, then drive over the unemphatic landscape of the Great Plains to my wife in Denver.

In the early spring Abbe and I take a vacation to St. Thomas in the U.S. Virgin Islands, perhaps for no other reason than to contemplate the direction of our life together. We spend our days there on the fine flourlike beaches only to watch the implacable routine of the sun cross the salt-colored sky. Because of my photosensitive skin, I whiten myself with sunblock, cloak my head beneath a hat, my hands beneath gloves, and shield my eyes behind large insectlike sunglasses. But shortly after arriving on the small coral island, something strange happens. From day to day I feel the girth of my abdomen expanding. At first I don't mention anything to Abbe; we are here to forget for a little while, to immerse ourselves in hopefulness. The slow though inexorable deterioration of my heart is a subject we conspicuously ignore. But here lies my belly, cresting over my shorts while my feet and ankles swell out of my shoes. For two days I remain quietly terrified, but eventually even Abbe can't help but notice. I am thirty-four years old and we both suspect I am in congestive heart failure.*

It is a kind of panic in slow motion, a dread that runs so deep and thick I become paralyzed for a few days. I see now that I am dying, and late one night in our windowless hotel room I tell Abbe so. The disease is slowly surpassing the available technology. But she isn't hearing any of it; I am jumping to grandiose conclusions; it may not even be my heart at all. Her voice is peremptory and tinged with the hostile spirit of denial.

Eventually we leave St. Thomas for Miami where I call Michael Sarché and tell him what's happening, how my body is mutating into a gelatinous mass overnight. He listens patiently two thousand miles away, asks a series of questions, then comes to the same conclusion I have. This is the bloody handiwork of this disease. He prescribes Lasix, a powerful diuretic to shed the water weight, then tells me to see him first thing when I return.

Later in the week I ask rhetorically, "This is the beginning of the end, isn't it, Michael?"

He pulls the stethoscope from his ears and derisively shrugs his shoulders. "You're in congestive heart failure. We'll treat you with Lasix as we need to." The inflection in his voice is a meek attempt at reassurance. He remarks about the racket of my sick heart, the sound of a gallop between beats and reiterates that he has seen it all many times before. But all I hear is the flaccid tone of his voice, because this is what I choose to listen to. He cannot dismiss the air of dread.

"Am I dying, Michael?"

He draws a breath and begins to speak, choosing his words with particular care.

---

*A state in which the heart's ability to pump is no longer adequate, and as a result the body begins to retain fluid.

"Your condition is deteriorating, Bob. But, no, I wouldn't say you are dying. We still have several options at our command."

"When I was lying on that sunny beach I felt like I was dying. I felt like this disease was finally catching up with me."

I see Michael looking down at the floor. Suddenly he lifts his head and speaks.

"This disease is never going to just go away."

Because I have been in atrial fibrillation since my return, that afternoon we decide I should see a cardiac electrophysiologist, a superspecialist who knows all there is to know about the electrical activity of the heart. These people can be intimidating, even to other physicians, because to be one you must be, in a word, brilliant. This specialist recommends higher doses of amiodarone.

But as the higher doses accumulate in my body, I feel the slow, steady, glacial return of water to my belly and legs in spite of the diuretics. Moreover, my heart has continued its fluttering rhythm, the fibrillation that amiodarone is supposed to quell, and the symptoms return with such force that I feel I'll be dead within days. I am breathless in bed, as though my heart were laboring just to keep me alive while at rest, so the next day I call Dr. Sarché to tell him what I suspect: the amiodarone is killing me; it's causing the congestive heart failure. After having given me a new life for nearly two years, for some reason it's contributing to the symptoms.

So I call around the country to cardiologists whom I know to be experts on amiodarone, and find one doctor who claims to have witnessed the drug causing heart failure in a patient of his. With that I go to Dr. Sarché's office and ask him if it would be all right to stop the amiodarone cold, and he says he doesn't have a problem with it so long as I understand we are treading unknown waters.

But due to the properties of the drug, particularly its extraor-

dinary half-life, my skin retains its smoky blue hue, and the fibrillation hangs in my chest with tenacious resolve for several
weeks. Psychiatric residency training is scheduled to begin on
the first of the month, and as the window of time draws to a
close, the residue of amiodarone retreats from my body, taking
with it the toxic side effects and the blue tint in my skin. Just
days before my residency begins I feel my heart finally growing
sure of itself, and the fibrillation ceases. But I now understand
my physical reality will always prevent me from extinguishing
the psychological symptoms of depersonalization and panic entirely. My prognosis would be different if these symptoms were
the result of neurotic conflicts, but in my case they are an appropriate response to the daily threats to my life. I can only attempt
to manage them as best I can.

Psychiatry training brings unexpected comforts. I am formally learning the science of the mind, plumbing its murky
depths, charting the altered landscape. I understand that it lives
a life of its own, and I recognize my unique insight into its secret
nature. The director of residency training knows me too; he is
Dr. Jay Scully, the large, soft-spoken man who placed me under
Dr. Gaensbauer's care ten years ago.

The year before psychiatric residency training began I saw Dr.
Scully again as my personal psychiatrist. In his small quiet office
I told him the long gritty tale of the last ten years and its harrowing aftermath. Peripherally I saw how the tale affected him.
Small tears coalesced in the folds of his eyes; he uttered audible
gasps as his pen rested in his large limp hand. As the story drew
to a close, he said with grave certainty, "You know, your affliction is post-traumatic stress disorder, PTSD—what all these
Vietnam vets are being diagnosed with."

The voice was an epiphany with the effect of a vast landscape
suddenly being lit up by a flash of lightning. After a short medi-

tative pause, he began again: "Your story can be interpreted as a metaphor for warfare. What you have is old-fashion shell shock."

But once psychiatry residency formally commenced in July of 1985, we mutually decided our meetings should come to a close since otherwise Dr. Scully would be my psychiatrist and boss as the new director of residency. And at the time I had never felt more emotionally solid, in part because I had further isolated the problem. During residency I first came in contact with Vietnam veterans who were misdiagnosed as schizophrenic just as I nearly was. Between us I sensed the immediate and strong bond of recognition. And through the course of psychiatry training I will read up on the nuances of what is now called post-traumatic stress disorder, or PTSD. But it is the secret history of the disease that defines it most poignantly; it is the unspoken history of our culture of warfare.

In a handout from a medical school professor I came across an explanation of PTSD as it arose in military combat. I have since been unable to locate its source. It is an excellent summary of the history of PTSD.

During much of the nineteenth century, soldiers suffering from PTSD were accused of cowardice, which in turn was stigmatized as a character defect. This supposed moral taint first manifested itself in trembling, a symptom that was followed by "symptoms" of desertion: running and hiding. (I recognized this in my own agoraphobia ten years ago, when I couldn't leave my apartment.) The trouble with this diagnosis, however, was that it did not explain why so many highly decorated soldiers often showed signs of severe emotional stress.

The term *nostalgia* appeared during the Civil War. It was applied to those who yearned for home after long exposure to combat. Nostalgia was a form of depression in which the soldier could think only of his home and his desire to be there. The concept of nostalgia recognized for the first time that brave fighters as well as their less courageous comrades could suffer from the identical affliction.

The term *shell shock* appeared during the first world war, which was to a large extent a fixed war of attrition fought with artillery. In 1917 it was accepted that fear manifested itself before and during combat, but surrendering to it was labeled as cowardice.

In 1921, Ferenczi, Abraham, Simmel, and Jones, all disciples of Freud, came out with "Psychoanalysis and the War Neurosis," in which they described treating German soldiers with hypnosis, relieving traumatic symptoms much in the same way I had experienced relief with desensitization therapy.

In the early days of World War II, American forces experienced extremely high psychiatric casualty rates. A new term arose: *war neurosis,* side by side with "shell shock." Nonetheless, Major General Paul Howley, Chief Surgeon of the U.S. Army, stated that the basic cause of psychoneurosis was "insufficient courage." It is noteworthy that psychoneurosis was not a problem in the Russian army—a fact that no psychiatrist could account for. The answer is brutally simple: the communists executed those found guilty of cowardice. This draconian approach may have been in General Patton's mind when he announced late in the war that soldiers who refused combat due to "war neurosis" would be accused of cowardice.

After World War II, neuropsychiatrist, psychoanalyist, and author Roy Grinker wrote that "No matter how strong, normal, or stable a man might be, if the stress is sufficient for that individual's threshold, he will develop a war neurosis."

It is difficult to discuss the role of the war neurosis in the Vietnam War. For one thing, the average age of the World War II GI was twenty-six; in Vietnam it was nineteen. There was no buddy system in Vietnam, just a one-year rotation. Vietnam was a civil war, with heavy and visible participation of the civilian population, and the war was not supported by many Americans. These factors, and others, made return to a normal life especially hard for many U.S. veterans.

As I read this I come to understand it as my private allegory. Depersonalization, the strange dissociative state during which I experienced feelings of unreality and detachment from my environment, as described by Dr. Roth, is a common symptom of PTSD. My history has been a kind of theater of war. With the gentle guidance of Dr. Scully, I see my project is to uncover the elaborate metaphor, like an archaeologist unearthing and interpreting an ancient Roman battlefield.

27

Late one night after returning to our dark and quiet home, I find Abbe curled up on the sofa, her eyes weary and reluctant. I sit down in the quiet pale light then gently ask her what's the matter. In a voice both tentative and stern she tells me Jessica has had a stroke and has just been discharged from the ICU at the University of California San Francisco Hospital. The room is hushed. I ask a few basic questions then go to the phone and call her myself. Her voice confirms the news; she is disoriented, searching for words that once came to her in brilliant, lucid strands of thought. This voice that was fluent in five languages is now a bland mumble, uncertain of itself, grim with fear and confusion. Eight years ago she underwent a kidney transplant after juvenile diabetes had destroyed her own kidneys, and now the donor organ is being rejected by the invisible forces of her immune system. And apparently her death is all but imminent as the immunosuppressants, the drugs that hold her body at bay and keep it from attacking her new kidney, are suspected of having caused the stroke. With or without the drugs she will die. The conversation is simple but convoluted as she struggles to make meager points. When we say our final goodbye I feel a surge of tears overwhelming my voice.

•   •   •

Jessica and I share more than a common ancestry; we share a common history and fate. In tiny increments my heart slowly deteriorates, yet Michael Sarché keeps me alive and functioning through the course of residency training. In May 1988, after four years of training, I am handed another diploma. At age thirty-eight I become a psychiatrist.

As though by the force of gravity I move from graduation to work at the V.A. Hospital down the street consulting and treating the most troubled Vietnam veterans. I become part of a team made up of professors of psychiatry and a psychopharmacologist whose focus is primarily on the post-traumatic stress disorder that these men suffer from. And I am the front lines, the treating physician, the one these men come to trust. There is a natural camaraderie. I also open a private practice where I see an astounding number of people with severe personality disorders who have hauntingly similar symptoms of depersonalization and derealization. Oftentimes from physical, sexual, or even emotional abuse, they describe to me how their consciousness dissociates or breaks down into its component parts. They too experience flashbacks, suffer amnesia, feelings of unreality and not being of their body or a part of their environment. What I glean from their stories is a theory that all sources of trauma encompass experiences taken from all walks of life. I rethink earlier notions: one does not have to live beyond the realm of common human experience to suffer as I have. Psychological neglect and lack of appropriate nurturing I see can sprout the same emotional virus in children, and perhaps it is this lack of nurturing that is the common trauma of the human race. It is a grandiose thought, one of those ponderous large truths.

•   •   •

Those afflicted with serious genetic illness all share the common dilemma of whether or not to have children. There is the special contingency of guilt that comes with mere speculation. An agonizing dialectic develops through the years that pits nature against mathematics. Any child I father has a one in two chance of inheriting IHSS, which makes fatherhood a kind of roulette with genetics. Discussions surface late at night and in the early morning, gentle philosophical arguments concerning the benchmark that demarcates when life is and is not worth living. More small truths emerge, modest convictions. My life has been worthwhile, I would rather have been than not. Even a child with IHSS stands to be useful to and happy in this world, just as I feel I have been.

In the rainy fall of 1988 we make a conscious decision to go ahead, to make a child with or without all the potential for flaws, and love it for all its unique imperfection. Then we get right down to it, and a month later I come home late in the evening to have Abbe announce she is pregnant. We talk in the kitchen, reassuring each other we have done the right thing, and without being entirely aware of it, I devour every perishable food within my reach. After a few minutes, Abbe pauses and stares at me in bewilderment.

"Bob, look at you."

"What?"

"You've eaten an apple, a banana, most of the pasta salad . . ."

We stare rather solemnly into each other's eyes.

"I'm happy, I'm scared. We did the right thing, didn't we?" I say.

"I know we did."

During the Christmas break that year, Abbe and I take a ski vacation to Steamboat Springs where my father owns a condominium. While there I discover a lifestyle I could get used to. One evening at the beginning of our stay I am asked by local friends if I would see a couple who is having marital troubles. So for the next ten days I ski during the day, slowly and carefully, but I ski nonetheless, and in the evenings I see this couple. The routine is invigorating though perhaps a little unrealistic to imagine as a lifestyle for me. But before heading back to Denver, back to the gray urban streets and perpetual hum of a large western town, I ask an internist at the local hospital if he thinks there is a need for a psychiatrist in the area. Definitely yes, he says. So I make arrangements to drive up every Friday to work with patients, and within but a few weeks I am in Steamboat Springs three days a week seeing these referrals.

Through the hot spring and summer months Abbe carries our baby to term and on July 31, 1989, gives birth to a big baby boy. We name him Max Jacob Pensack. What I deliver with my own hands is a healthy eight-pound nine-ounce baby, and with his weight in my arms I carry about a new peacefulness. A circle closes. At night Abbe will awake to crying and bring our son between us in bed, then, together we coo him to sleep. Eventually Abbe and I will join him in a world of infant dreams, as a family.

As the practice in Steamboat Springs continues to grow it becomes more and more realistic to simply move there, migrate to where I am needed most. To some these plans appear outlandish, particularly those close to me. My heart is gradually failing, yet my anxiety continues to fade. I have a new son, and now want to move deep into the mountains, away from the support and security of a large metropolitan hospital. But all these considerations are surmountable with modern conveniences, and besides, it's something both Abbe and I have always wanted to do. After all, I am not long for this world. Such knowledge goes a long way toward an erratic life.

In Steamboat we live in what appears to visitors to be a Swiss chalet in a shallow valley known as Strawberry Park. The property borders the National Forest lands of Buffalo Pass and lies just two miles from the old town. At night the sky glows above the city lights like a luminous pink parasol. During the summer and fall months I see patients during the day and read through their case histories at night, and in the winter I try to ski whenever feeling up to it. But the heart grows intolerant. There is the familiar heady sense that something is about to happen. From month to month I feel the gradual flagging of the heart, and suspect with a sickening dread that those options Dr. Sarché spoke of are dwindling.

Then one quiet evening the phone rings and Richard's panicked voice stammers on the other end. He has been in the hospital for four days in San Francisco after an acute episode of ventricular tachycardia that nearly killed him. Then for good measure, the attending physician gave him Inderal, the same drug I was on years ago when my heart was much stronger. The drug was administered to correct Richard's tachycardia, and sent him into cardiogenic shock by making an extremely weak heart even weaker. He is no longer critical, he now explains, but you wouldn't guess it by his weak and terrified voice.

The following day I fly out to San Francisco to be with him and help his young family along. His sixteen-year-old son, Benjamin, Richard tells me as he lies back in bed, has been recently diagnosed with IHSS. His eyes are glassy pools of hopelessness and defeat as he says this. Our baneful legacy has now reached my nephew. The news affects us similarly as I now think of Max, lying in his crib at home with a one-in-two chance of inheriting my heart. A prepared piano, an invisible illness, memory of my blood.

While there the preliminaries to the unimaginable take place. Richard researches the various heart-transplant programs in the area, because now it is all too clear that he will need a new heart if he is to survive. There are no other options. In the Bay Area there are three transplant programs, but the most convenient for Richard is Pacific Presbyterian Hospital, which is run by Dr. Donald Hill. Dr. Hill is guardedly reassuring. Yes, Richard will need a new heart for long-term survival, and no, it shouldn't be a long wait for a donor. Transplantation is another brave new world of medicine.

Of the 2.2 million people who will die in America in the coming year, Richard needs one of them to do so somewhere in his vicinity. This person must be his blood type, approximate size, and die in such a manner as not to damage his or her heart. But most important, brain death must occur first, as it inevitably did with Jessica, to allow for the retrieval or harvest of organs. Of those 2.2 million people, however, only four thousand will actually donate their organs. Every thirty minutes another patient is added to the national registry for organs of one type or another. The bottom line is that the arithmetic doesn't add up and thousands of people die every year waiting. Richard knows all of this, he knows it's a game of chance, but it's the only game in town. With heart and liver transplantation, the numbers are especially grim, as 25 percent of those waiting on the list will die before a donor heart is procured. But once an appropriate organ is found, the odds of short-term survival rise dramatically, with 85 percent of the patients surviving their first year, and 75 percent surviving for five years. The ten-year numbers still aren't available due to the newness of the technology.

During the 1970s a Swiss immunologist by the name of Jean Borel found a fungus in a soil sample that had some remarkable qualities, most notably that it was capable of suppressing the specific part of the body's immune system, the T-cell lymphocytes, that attack transplanted organs. The derivative of this fungus, cyclosporine, approved by the FDA in 1983, is a drug all organ-transplant patients take for the rest of their lives. It can be said that this man, Jean Borel, is responsible for saving the lives of hundreds of thousands of people, possibly my brother included.

Toward the end of the week Richard is formally listed and given a beeper, then once his condition is stabilized, I head back to Steamboat, to my practice and young family, and await the news that a donor heart has been found. While home my own heart deteriorates, almost as though in imitation of Richard's. I talk with Dr. Sarché on the phone in Denver and he asks me to come down so that its performance can be evaluated. What I want to know is if a heart transplant is in my immediate future. He has me climb aboard a treadmill, and my deterioration is obvious. He then refers me to the University Hospital to be evaluated by the cardiologist in charge of transplant medicine. With a degree of delight, the cardiologist, Dr. JoAnn Lindenfeld, tells me transplantation is too radical a move at this stage of my illness. Though I knew this would be the answer, I wanted to hear someone in transplant medicine say it. I don't try to conceal my faint traces of relief.

A few weeks later while I am immersed in a deep sleep the phone rings at 2:30 in the morning, and again it is Richard's agitated voice. A silent moment passes to allow me to separate dream from reality as the voice penetrates the static.

". . . Bob . . . Bob . . . I just got a call from the hospital . . . They've got a heart for me . . ."

His speech is rambling, broken by archaic Hebrew idioms.

". . . I've called Dad and told him . . . they have a heart . . . *baruch Hashem* . . ."

I say something without hearing it. Then, "It's happening?"

". . . It's happening, Bob. I've got to go now, things are hurried."

"I love you, Richard. I'll be on the first plane to San Francisco."

"You've been a good brother, Bob . . ." And the line goes dead.

The next time I see Richard is with my father as his gurney is rushed out of the OR suite. I touch his cooled flesh as he rounds the corner, surrounded by doctors and nurses commanding everyone to get out of the way. Then for the next four days, Richard's body is slowly raised from the dead, the invisible forces of his body warded away by the mysterious drug derived from Jean Borel's fungus, along with a cocktail of others, including a modern version of ALG, Starzl's drug, called Atgam. His heart takes to him as it sustains his body day after day, that precious flesh of another's flesh, that gift of goodwill distilled in the blood of another.

As Richard's body heals itself amid the calamity of monitors and the most sophisticated medical technology known to man, I think of the parallel though separate courses our lives have taken. I suppose the counterpart of this process to the faithful would be called prayer, though I have difficulty thinking of it as such. Richard would certainly call it prayer. He has drifted to faith through the years, whereas I have clung to the science of the mind. When I imagine Richard I see his long dense beard, his *tzitzis,* the holy cloth that he dresses in every morning before pulling on his street clothes. I see Richard studying his Torah, I see him boarding an airliner with his former wife Linda, and son, Benjamin, and flying to Israel where he brings himself and his family closer to the faith of our mother and father. I picture the concern laden in his eyes as I tell him about a cardiac arrest of mine, and his saying *baruch Hashem,* blessed be God, like a reflex of love as he places a hand on my shoulder. Then I think of the mathematics that await him, the ambush of chance.

But miraculously he recovers, as though by the will of his God. When Richard emerges from the small death of Lazarus, his ancient predecessor, the ancestor of all transplant patients, I stay at his bedside with the family until he is actually able to sit up and even take a few steps. For the next few days I come to know other families in the lounge. And slowly it occurs to me why we are all here at the same time. One donor has given life to all our relatives, we are all bound by blood as one donor has given a liver, a heart, two kidneys, a pancreas, bone marrow, eyes, skin, everything there was to give. It occurs to me we are all family—*every man is a peece of the continent, a part of the maine.*

28

A new heart is inescapable, it is the only exit. When I return to Steamboat I can't walk the two flights of stairs to my office without stopping every few steps to allow my heart to recover. The bloating of water weight returns, my girth deepens with alarming suddenness, which I counter with more diuretics that cloak the symptoms of congestive heart failure. Every day I announce to Abbe when I return home from work utterly exhausted, "I need a new heart," and she responds with a glib, "You'll die." She simply wants me alive. If I can't get off the couch, but can live till I'm eighty, then that would be just fine. But that isn't the case, and she secretly knows this. She knows I will be dead soon without a transplant, which is what she can't bring herself to address.

The following year Abbe announces she is again pregnant, and in May of 1991 gives birth to a baby girl whom we name Miriam Rose Pensack. Again, I deliver her with my own hands. There is the same internal argument, the same cruel apprehension and hope, but afterward we decide this will be it. We are at once grateful for what appears to be a healthy baby girl, and terrified that she may possess a heart with intrinsic flaws that will remain camouflaged until adolescence.

And the slow and steady failure of my own heart only heightens these misgivings. The following winter while in Florida I again find myself calling Michael Sarché from a hotel room, describing with raging alarm the abrupt metamorphosis of this gelatinous body. While lying in bed I struggle for breath as though drowning in my own fluid; mere walking is fantastically exhausting. I tell him I'm dying; he tells me to hurry home.

Two days later when he puts me on a treadmill I notice his eyes are sullen, almost grave. Right away they fall to the floor as my thick and bloated legs toil upon the conveyor belt. The hum of the machine driven by these puffy legs hardly makes an audible sound before it dies in the echo of the clinic. The legs slow to a stop; the rasp of my breath fills the room. I look over at Michael, his eyes fixed on the grid of linoleum seams. There are no voices, only murky sounds, the sonorous echoes of the subterranean. Then our eyes meet.

"Bob, it's time . . ."

"I know."

His eyes well up, he tells me that he loves me, then I too cry.

After meeting with Dr. Lindenfeld and another cardiologist by the name of Dr. Bristow, I return to Steamboat. Moments after breathlessly entering the door I take Abbe into my arms, and as though echoing the haunting words of Michael Sarché, I say, "Abbe, it's time."

The following week, Abbe, Max, Miriam and I drive back to Denver to sit down with the three main cardiologists in transplant medicine at the University Hospital and are told what lies in store for me. Much of it I am already familiar with, but the protocol and treatment for receiving a donor heart is so vast and comprehensive in its effect on one's life that I don't think any one person on the staff has all the answers. What I ask for is the bottom line.

"How long do I have without this transplant?" I ask Dr. Bristow.

His manner is casual. "Twelve, eighteen months."

Abbe's hand swims over to my knee, then our eyes meet.

Like Richard, I am to be placed on the national computer list maintained by the United Network of Organ Sharing (UNOS). The names on the list are prioritized according to the criteria of urgency of need, length of time listed, and blood and tissue types, as well as the vicinity in which organs become available relative to those who need them. At the University Hospital, the success rate is considerably higher than the national average, which is due largely to Dr. Lindenfeld and a surgeon by the name of Dr. Dave Campbell. From the beginning this surgeon is mysterious, almost a mythical character who lives in my imagination as the hero of a Homeric tale.

Through the course of my next several meetings he is never present, seemingly always busy with a transplant on a child or another adult. In my imagination he remains unintentionally aloof, burdened with the business of saving human lives.

Then one day as I come out of clinic, I am told that Dr. Campbell is waiting for me outside in the hallway. With a degree of excitement I step outside, anxious to see this creature who spends his day with his hands in the chests of others. But when I look about there is no one around but a young man in a World War II bomber jacket, surgical greens and sneakers without any socks. Eventually a nurse comes with a patient dragging an IV pole behind her as they work their way down the hall, but no one who looks very doctorly. Finally the young man who appears to be a medical student approaches me and asks if I'm Dr. Pensack, then introduces himself as Dave Campbell. For a moment I'm beside myself.

That afternoon we visit together. I ask him about the surgical procedure itself, what's involved with the recovery, how long I'll wait for a heart. He is haltingly candid, and tells me there's no telling how long. He also tells me I don't need to move to Denver, that he'd personally come pick me up in a plane if that's what the circumstances called for. His manner portrays a man utterly without the entrapments of professionalism, a mere human being.

But I make the move back to Denver, if only because of the imperious advice of Dr. Bristow and my own sense of security. And three weeks after having been given a beeper I receive a call from Dr. Lindenfeld just after sitting down to dinner with my family in our new apartment.

"Don't eat dinner, Bob," she says. "We might have a heart for you."

Time is arrested.

Finally I stammer, "When will you know if it's a go?"

"About an hour. Stay calm, and don't get your hopes up."

I find myself growing euphoric, the adrenaline roiling in my blood at the prompting of fear. I shadow-box about the apartment while I wait for the phone to ring again. The hour passes, then another half hour, and another fifteen minutes. Forty-five minutes after the anticipated call, the enthusiasm of the household begins to leak. Hope is bled away, my body fatigues as the adrenaline fades, and finally the phone does ring. Earlier I had situated the phone at the center of the dining room table, poised it in a kind of ceremony. Now, as it rings, the brassy cry of its bell growing more and more portentous, I know it shouldn't be answered. It is not in the rhythm of good luck, if it was a go they would have called when they said they would. The phone only bears bad news.

"Bob?" the voice asks.

"Yes."

"I'm sorry, Bob."

"I know, JoAnn."

"The heart's better suited for someone else."

"I figured as much."

So begins a long walk through a dark corridor. I soon learn to manage feelings of impending doom in this universe over which I have no control. After the first false alarm, months pass as my heart keeps a desultory pace that seems to slowly wind down like the spent coil spring of a clock. At night I watch the reflection of the moon swing across the wooden floor in a pool of milky light while Abbe sleeps beside me, waking from time to time and pleading for me to get some rest. But night and day, consciously and unconsciously, I wait for the phone to ring or the beeper to sound its alarm. And they never do.

Through the grapevine of the transplant team at the hospital I discover the heart I was denied that night had gone to a man by the name of Ken Poirier from Craig, Colorado, a small mining town just west of Steamboat Springs. I ask Karin Keller, the transplant coordinator, if I could visit with the man, and she tells me I may, but that I shouldn't mention that his was the heart I didn't get. "Of course not," I say, amazed she thought she had to mention it.

When I meet him he seems alert, though he has the telltale "moonface," the puffiness of facial features caused by the steroids which assist in subduing the immune system. He is cheerful, still in command of his sense of humor, something I would imagine is difficult to retain. He tells me he was listed for an incredible seventeen months, certain toward the end that he would die before he received a heart. Then he reassures me I won't have to wait that long, and I tell him I'd better not because Dr. Bristow estimated this heart had a year to a year and a half left. We talk for a few minutes about our mutual home, and our mutual longing to return there, then I leave, sad, quiet and jealous. As I descend in the white noise of the elevator, I visualize his sanguine eyes, his expression of visceral satisfaction as he makes distant plans.

The next day I receive a call from John Ritota who tells me

about a man he met in Florida who has recently received a donor heart. He reminds John of me, he says, and I really need to call him.

When I call this man, Jimmy Tinnesz, he tells me his incredible story of how he was stationed in the Persian Gulf just prior to Desert Storm, and how he contracted a virus which slowly destroyed his heart. Perhaps he ate some bad fish, he says. He is a religious man I gather from his references to Christ, faith and his love for God and His world. We speak with an extraordinary ease and immediacy as we share stories of trauma, hopelessness and resiliency. Then toward the end of the conversation he invites me down to Florida to stay with him after I get the call and have recovered from the surgery.

The weather turns hot through the summer, the distilled atmosphere allowing the sun to bear down on the pavement of the city. On the Fourth of July Abbe and I take the children to Cherry Creek Reservoir to soak ourselves. Though I'm not strong enough to swim, I can float like an immense beach ball. On this bright summer day the mood is ominous on the beach. Abbe and the kids shift sand into castles and moats while I float on my back and gaze into the empty blue. My ears are submerged, my eyes blinking away lapping rifts, the horizon of water and crown of my nose surrounding the sky. I feel the gentle lifting and sinking of my body with the rhythm of breath. Then I inhale and sink into the cool blue as though in a rehearsal for a resurrection. After resurfacing, I make my way to shore and breathlessly trudge toward Abbe as she comes at me with a towel.

"You want to go back to Steamboat?" I ask as she whirls the towel about my shoulders.

She smiles and wipes away an intricate pattern of sweat beads from her brow.

"Only if it won't kill you."

"Nothing has yet."

So Abbe packs through the night, and the following day we wind through the high and cool mountains to our home in Steamboat. We settle in once again, rearrange our life of provisional survival, tell ourselves it won't be long now—all against the backdrop of a failing heart.

CROSS-SECTION OF DESIRE

29

I've taken to sitting back and watching the wind make waves of the wheatfields. Sunlight disappears then quickly reappears from behind small swiftly moving cumulus clouds cruising in a perfect lateral plane down the valley. The view calms, keeps the mind in check. Yet every now and then fear slowly rises up and settles high up near the chest. Within the roar of the wind, I hear the wheat seething as if the countryside lay gripped by some impalpable anger, the dry ripe kernels rustling against each other in a sea of gold. I look away before the noise fills my head, my mind seizes with panic.

Abbe lays a hand on my thigh; her lips crease into a smile as though she has sensed the rush rising up in me. She then returns her attention to the road, her eyes scanning the landscape behind the sunglasses.

Soon we're on the interstate, descending into the phosphorescent lights of Denver dominating the horizon. Once again we're in city traffic, jockeying for position in the fast lane, once again we're pulling into the familiar parking lot of the hotel near the hospital. I now see that sheer familiarity with the urban setting has cast a pall of general doubt. Here I am again.

That night neither Abbe nor I sleep restfully. Murmured conversations surface in the midst of the darkness, followed by silent restlessness, then another weary dialogue. In the morning as she emerges from the shower she finds me with a cup of coffee and another heady book whose narrator has renounced god, this time Elie Wiesel's *Night,* an account of the Holocaust. Abbe is one of the few who tolerates my need for depressing subject matter. I am only good at denial when feeling well; otherwise I want a clear view of a dark future, to swaddle myself in hopelessness.

As Abbe dresses before the bathroom mirror, I tell her she might as well remain poolside while I admit myself, as working my way through the bureaucracy will take hours. She whimsically agrees, but says she won't be lounging. She recites a mental list of errands to be run as she coasts a comb through her wet hair. I get my dop kit together while she calls Steamboat Springs to check on the kids. Apparently the weather there has deteriorated with snow predicted above nine thousand feet. I take my bags to the car, muttering as I make baby steps toward the carport, "A week before Labor Day. Jesus Christ, Labor Day." This makes it an eight-month wait.

The day is intensely bright, the trees lit with a bright yellow. A premature fall. The car slowly weaves through the students as they cross the street between the hospitals, clinics and university buildings, until the hospital looms over the treetops. The sight of the building itself is enough to conjure ambivalent feelings, that familiar tingle of hope and fear. Though I've had a catheter threaded into my heart dozens of times, it's something one never gets used to. The puncturing of flesh never fails to startle, just as the invasion of steel and plastic never fails to leave the mind quivering with fear. Pain can become exhausting simply because you never get used to it. I ponder this thought as we drive.

Abbe drops me off within the shade of the breezeway over the front entrance. She reassures me it's all about to happen for us, then kisses my lips, my forehead. As I head down the narrow hallway old acquaintances simply nod or make brief small talk. Eventually I get to the small waiting area where I take a number to get my blood drawn and give a urine sample. A Korean girl with poor English finally calls my number and greets me by bowing slightly as if she hasn't been fully assimilated into American culture. After she has applied a rubber tourniquet then missed my vein twice, I tell her I'm a doctor and ask if I can do it myself. She blushes faintly at her failure, unaware that my mindless veins are privy to the conspiracy of needles. Soon dark vermilion flows into the cylinder as she looks on. The chamber is filled, my arm patched, then she hands me a dingy plastic urine-sample cup stained with use. This is easy. Urine, unlike blood, is bountiful when on diuretics.

I head upstairs to the EKG lab, then admissions, then to a pre-surgery waiting area where someone has sent me anticipating a long wait before I can get into the cath lab. I change into the hospital garb and flirt with the young nurse on duty. Finally a nurse I recognize from the cath lab appears at the end of the long empty room.

"We're ready for you, Dr. Pensack," she says, smoothing her greens with her small hands.

Once in the cath lab I climb onto the surgical table myself, take off my shirt, and the nurse asks me about my musical taste.

"How about Eric Clapton?"

"During a heart cath?"

"Too stimulating? Might induce a panic attack?"

The doctors come in wearing lead aprons while she scans the left side of the radio dial for a classical music station. Their voices are quick and terse.

"How are you, Bob?" Dr. Groves, the head cath surgeon, asks.

"Seldom well. Just waiting for this Swan."*

I close my eyes for a brief moment, try to relax, take a few slow rhythmic breaths in an attempt to dilute the intolerable feeling of vulnerability. They pull the sterile blue surgical drape over

---

*A Swan-Ganz catheter monitors pressures in the heart.

my head and ask me to look away. Though I can't see, I can hear them preparing the local anesthetic, the clack of surgical steel, the sound of liquid compressed through hypodermic needles.

Soon I feel the violent pinch of the needle into the trunk of my neck, then the initial tiny incision is made into the jugular. I feel warm blood spill onto my skin. I close my eyes again, take more thorough breaths, and go to some other place: in bed with my wife, a swift and clear mountain river, the blond sand of a vast beach in St. Martin; I visualize myself effortlessly running up the hill to our house. My eyes flutter, and I see the surreal sky-blue light of the surgical drape.

"Okay. You're going to feel a little pressure now," an anonymous voice announces.

I feel the Swan floating down my neck, and with it comes the overwhelming grip of claustrophobia. Suddenly something feels wrong. An eerie movement high up in my chest.

"It's not going down right," I hear myself say. "It's in my innominate vein." The pressure increases, filling my neck.

"That's all right. You're going to feel a little pressure," the same anonymous voice mumbles.

"It's going through my innominate, I can feel it. Now it's going up the other jugular, damn it," I say, feeling the Swan float beneath my Adam's apple.

"You're going to feel a little pressure."

"Take a look. You'll see it's not right."

They pull the fluoroscope over me, still skeptical, then see on the screen what I see in my mind's eye. The Swan finally retreats a little, then is again floating toward the heart. I mentally follow its course through the vena cava, into the right atrium, right ventricle, the pulmonary artery. I tell myself to think like a soldier, to live in the moment with no past or future. Only present. Suppress the imagination, shut off the living movie in my head. The pressure of the Swan floating down the jugular, the cold water thrust into the atrium, the chill filling my chest—the sensations aren't so painful as they are eerie and threatening.

Every now and then the Swan touches the chamber walls, causing my heart to skip a beat, a compensatory pause before resuming its regular pattern. A dizzy sensation washes across my forehead, yet I'm in control. I know what's going on. Then it happens again and again in quick succession. I tell myself to stay cool, to go to yet another place, to blot out the pictures of cadavers from the days of medical school. I tell myself I am one mean son of a bitch.

"I'm having PCVs,* lots of them," I say. The voice is distant, without resonance.

"It's all right. That's normal."

My heart shies from the catheter as the rigid plastic tickles the muscle. But explanations don't put me at ease. I've seen things go wrong in the cath lab. It's easy to underestimate the potential for mishap. Any direct line to the heart is fraught with danger. The potential for devastating infection, heart attack, arrhythmia, or puncturing the heart wall is always there. The procedure is no less bizarre and seemingly barbaric than something dreamt by a diseased mind, the mind of Dr. Frankenstein, Dr. Moreau. Yet my tentative future lies within the sleepless walls of this hospital, in the cold hands of masked surgeons. I am merely a purveyor of nameless static rage.

---

*Premature ventricular contractions, or an irregular heartbeat caused by contact between the catheter and the heart wall.

30

For three days I wait in the ICU for a heart that doesn't come. Yet small consolations lie in wait like glittering rhinestones in a vast rough. Apparently my heart likes Dobutamine, the drug that entices it to squeeze harder. Physically I'm feeling better, thanks to large doses of the fancy pharmaceutical that drips from an IV bag into my arm. But I'm tired of being hurt. What frightens me most is the suspicion that I don't want this heart. Not now. I don't want to be stuck or cut, much less pried open, anymore. And living three days with a catheter in my neck is like getting my teeth cleaned when viewed against having my heart dissected and another one sewn in. The ambivalence is unsettling. I ask myself academic questions: Do I want to live after all? Would I not be better off returning to Steamboat and letting IHSS run its bloody course? Does this heart house a coward shrinking from pain? Instinct tells me I want to live, that I'll do what it takes.

While cardiologists and nurses check blood pressures deep within my heart, I hold court to a steady line of friends from medical school, answer phone calls, read—all with this spike in my neck. Simple motions are now difficult or impossible. My head no longer rotates, as twisting tugs the catheter line. I depend on peripheral vision.

On the third day Dr. Bristow leads a troupe of young resident cardiologists into the room where they silently shuffle into a semicircle around my bed. Their faces all hold slight variations of a pasty-white color, their eyes distant and vacant, not seeing yet absorbing what is said. No doubt they have all been awake through the night. Suddenly Bristow places his palms together and says:

"Well. We're going to transplant you."

I know of his penchant for fantastic statements, but he has my heart pounding off my chest nevertheless.

"We're going to keep you here through the Labor Day weekend to see if anything happens," he says, his eyes focused on my chin.

"Okay," I say, drawing deep breaths. "So this is it. I'm in the hospital for good now." To be in the hospital through a holiday weekend is serious business. This means I'm their man. This would make me status one, at the very top of the list in the entire state.

"For good, Bob."

The next day they move me from the ICU to the medical floor where I'm attached to fewer machines. The room is like any other hospital room, with regular nurses and a single heart monitor that produces a soft steady beep. Here I feel more like a living creature, less lonesome and frightened. Here beside me the broad arched leaves of a rubber plant given to me by a friend, poised to receive sunlight, on the chair a book is splayed, a tale of horror and suffering and survival I can identify with. These small things fill me with an exquisite joy. My only wish is the assurance that I may live among them indefinitely. I secretly know there is no telling when this heart will arrive.

Sometimes while lying awake during the dark and quiet hour before dawn I wonder if it's to come at all. My roommate, Jerry, a man in his late fifties, wasn't accepted on the transplant list due to the advanced stage of his heart disease. His cardiologist neglected to refer him for transplantation several years ago while his health was still adequate to undergo the surgery. If they were to transplant him today, he would die on the table. Now he's gaunt, frail, his translucent wrists showing gray streaks of veins. He quietly saunters about the ward, pulling his IV carriage and oxygen tank like the ball and chain of a condemned man. Though his condition has nothing in common with mine, he is something of a specter, a living ghost of what I'll become if this new heart doesn't find me in time.

I explain his condition to Abbe, whispering his dark prognosis so that he doesn't overhear while resting just beyond the curtain. "I'm a lucky fellow," I tell her.

Labor Day arrives on cat's feet, bringing with it a dense fog. The effect of Dobutamine has vanished with decreasing doses as they wean me off the drug. Apparently it has no residual effect. I've gained three pounds overnight and I get tired merely walking the halls. Weight gain means my heart is failing. If you take away the Dobutamine, I become bloated with water and tire easily.

To lift my spirits a nurse tells me I need to meet a man on seven west. A real inspiration, she repeats. Just four days ago he was transplanted and already he's walking around.

"He was joking about how sore he was," she says, lowering an eyebrow in a maternal way.

"I'll visit him tonight."

"He has this incredible attitude," she adds.

"I'll go up now if he's awake."

"I was just there. He's awake."

I climb out of bed, unplug the IV and drag the apparatus to the elevators and head to the transplant ward on the next floor. As I wait for the elevator doors to part, I sense a return of the same nervousness that accompanies anyone about to glimpse their future. One gets accustomed to the solace of ignorance. Above me in the transplant ward lies a man whose death has been postponed by the living tissue of the dead. But apprehension disperses as I walk down the brightly decorated halls of the transplant ward. This is the one ward in the hospital where they've made a visible effort at resembling a private hospital. Somebody has clearly worried over the wallpaper choice in matching it with the solidly laminated Formica counter at the front desk. The covers on the fluorescent lights are new, casting the fresh wax in a less severe brightness, not the pale yellow that throws a certain gloom down the other halls. The residents here have seen their share of gloom. Someone's good intentions are made clear. I trudge to the front desk and ask for Mr. Debey's room.

"Do you know him?" a nurse at the front desk asks.

"No, but I'm on the transplant list myself. I understand he was transplanted last Sunday night."

"He's an incredible man," she says. Her face is stern and serious.

"A nurse downstairs on the medical ward said he'd make me feel lucky," I say. As we talk, Mr. Debey takes on the power of myth in my mind.

"You know, he used to fly Air Force One for Eisenhower."

"He's sixty years old, right?"

"That's right," she says, slowly leading me down the hallway.

Mr. Debey is sitting up in bed watching college football when we enter. His shirt is off, displaying the telltale incision and staples down the sternum. He appears quite relaxed apart from being absorbed in the game. The nurse introduces me and his attention immediately snaps from the screen.

"I've heard a lot about you, Mr. Debey," I say. "You certainly look well."

He lifts his feet from the bed and leans over to shake my hand.

"I actually do feel okay. I'm not going to lie to you," he says, showing faint signs of discomfort. He's slightly short of breath, his face crimped as he shifts his weight about. "It wasn't no picnic."

"So you've been walking around already."

"Oh yeah. I'll tell you what, this heart feels like my own," he says, his gaze shifting about the room. "They told me it was a kid's down in New Mexico. A twenty-year-old heart."

I feel a pang of jealousy. I want a twenty-year-old heart. I want a heart just like Mr. Debey's.

"I'll be honest with you, though. It wasn't no picnic." His eyes continue to dart about the room as he speaks. "But the surgery was a breeze. Slept right through it."

"I certainly hope so," I say. I laugh, but notice he doesn't comprehend the humor in what he said.

"I'll be truthful, now. It wasn't no picnic when I woke up."

"I've had open heart surgery," I say, lifting my shirt to show my T-scar.

"Yep. It wasn't no picnic, was it?"

I remind myself that Mr. Debey is merely a little repetitious in the face of powerful medication with personality-distorting side effects, aside from the trauma of the transplant.*

"Do you like college football?" I ask.

"Oh yes. I do like football," he says as if citing a scientific fact.

"Would it be okay if I come up around two o'clock tomorrow and we watch the Buffs game together?"

"Oh, certainly, certainly."

I say goodbye and head back down to my room where I find Jerry resting there with the lights off. His wife sits beside him

---

*Transplant patients are generally given a regimen of three different immunosuppressant drugs, prednisone, cyclosporine and Imuran. Prednisone, a steroid, has the side effects of causing severe mood swings, agitation, irritability, and general emotional lability. In severe cases it has caused frank psychotic thinking, including paranoia and delusions.

reading a travel journal magazine within a crack of light shooting between a part in the drapes. I lie back, kick my feet up and try to read without success.

While staring up at the ceiling into the sanded tiles, trying to calm my mind, I hear Abbe's voice approaching from down the hallway greeting doctors, nurses and patients. She enters the room whispering, seeing the lights are off, the shades drawn. I immediately begin telling her about Mr. Debey's twenty-year-old heart and his remarkable recovery.

"He was transplanted only five days ago," I whisper.

"I heard he's sixty years old?"

"Yeah, but he's a little loose from the drugs."

"I suppose that's inevitable."

"Promise me you'll let me know when I'm that way."

We lie in bed together talking in hushed voices about what to do with the kids for the first few weeks after the transplant. I thrive on the language of certainty, speaking of the missing heart with a degree of urgency. Their daddy won't be able to pick them up, hold or play with them. We decide it would be best to keep them up in Steamboat while I'm convalescing as my withdrawal might give them cause to think I don't love them, or I don't want to be touched. I tell Abbe I'm ready to go back home, that I'm confident it will all happen with me lying there on the sofa just as soon as it will here in the hospital. It is rather pleasant lying in the cool and quiet darkness, speaking of hopeful matters.

At two o'clock the next day we head up to Mr. Debey's room. The game with Baylor is a blowout consistently interrupted by nurses and Mr. Debey's nebulous thinking patterns. I tell him I'm feeling better physically, but emotionally I'm down, I'm ready to go home, to be with the wife and kids. He lifts his hands, palms skyward, and says matter-of-factly, "They'll tell you when they have one."

"Well, I certainly hope so, Mr. Debey."

Abbe finds him charming, and we have an uplifting visit. I consider Mr. Debey the most audacious of men.

That evening a doctor from the lung-transplant team appears in the doorway. He introduces himself to Abbe, then says he has heard of me from doctors on the heart-transplant team. He says things are looking up, that these things inexplicably run in cycles. One week they'll get five or six donors, then they endure a four-month barren stretch.

"We got two hearts tonight," he says, his eyes smiling. "They sent one to Colorado Springs, the other they're transplanting downstairs tonight. Unfortunately they were both ABs and you're an A, right?"

Abbe and I nod.

"We could be on the crest of another cycle," he says. He smiles reassuringly then leaves.

"Well, those good intentions missed their mark," I say.

Abbe simply closes her eyes, her mouth gapes open.

While I lie awake in bed that night, my nurse Gwen comes in to check Jerry's vitals then my own. The hospital is still quiet since many patients were discharged during Labor Day. Gwen whispers hello as she passes in the dim light, then seeing that Jerry is resting, pulls a chair up beside my bed and asks about Max and Miriam.

"They're staying with friends."

"You look a little down."

"They're doing a heart downstairs, an AB. I'm ready to go home, heart or no heart."

"It'll happen," she whispers. We sit in the dark and whisper our conversation. I dwell on her voice, as it carries the soft steady melody of the deep south, the dignified tone of a Southern Baptist black woman. Georgia. She still calls me Dr. Pensack, though we've come to know each other well. I love her observance of small formalities. We sit together for half an hour or so until I feel my mind dozing. I hear her somnolent voice as I surface between opaque dreams into the room's suppressed light, then I submerge in sleep, a tangled web of dream and memory.

The following morning I awake to a ringing phone, happy that I've slept without awaking before dawn. Instead of answering it, I unplug the IV and head up to Mr. Debey's room where I find him shaving with a washbasin in his lap.

"Thought you were heading home," he says, glancing from a small mirror propped against a pillow.

"I'm leaving this afternoon, Mr. Debey. I wanted to see you before I leave," I say. My voice is oddly formal, as though I were addressing a rabbi.

He casually finishes shaving, wipes his face with a warm towel, then hoists himself off the bed.

"How about we head over to that lounge," he says, waving an index finger toward the door.

Together we make our way down the hall to the lounge where we sit among other transplant patients and their families. We talk about my disease and the disease he had before exchanging it for this new set of problems. He talks about his first biopsy after the transplant that yielded little rejection. He seems disinterested, his eyes wander about the room.

"I'll be honest with you. That first biopsy had me a little worried. I won't tell you it didn't," he says. His mouth appears strangely mobile, his jowls flaccid, exaggerating his southern drawl. I allow a little silence in deference to his anxiety that he bears with such equanimity.

Finally I ask the question. "Did you ever get depressed waiting for your heart?"

"Depressed? Well, now," he begins. His thoughts seem to have trailed off into confusion, so we sit in silence again while I wait for an appropriate opportunity to begin the conversation again. But just as I'm about to speak, his mind seems to snap back. He begins by telling me about a close business associate who died nearly twenty years ago, and a poor business deal that followed. I listen carefully, anticipating a circular argument or anecdote that requires a background, a vivid backdrop. Then the subject of depression drops away altogether, returning once his story spirals back to a series of false alarms from the transplant team. Apparently, several months ago he was called in for a new heart, given his first dose of cyclosporine and prednisone, sent to the OR and shaved. Once there he was anesthetized only to awake with no new heart, the organ having suffered some trauma in the accident or the harvest. For whatever reason, it was unusable.

Mr. Debey continues to talk, seemingly oblivious to my presence, about his extensive hospital experiences. He can't seem to stop talking. It is as if he feels the need to express every thought in his head, without any process of selection or priority. Whatever he thinks, no matter how insignificant, he says it. Eventually I lose track of the convoluted pattern, and tell him I need to be going.

"Back home, huh?"

"I miss my kids."

"Well. Better luck next time."

"I'm not a lucky man, Mr. Debey."

31

Outside it is October, early winter. The sky is snowing through two cones of floodlights above the living room windows. I lie reposed among the dim uneven shades, somewhere between three and four in the morning, watching the snow descend in spiraling tendrils and accumulate. An invisible train shunts through the distance, and is gone.

The silence is astounding. My wife and children sleep through the silent activity, while my mind is seized with insomnia. From time to time I move about the shadows like a ghost through the gray light until I become breathless and collapse in a heap into my chair before the window. I place a hand over my heart, feel its manic flutter gradually retreat into my chest.

These small hours are haunted, revisited by the living dead: Mr. Debey, Jerry, Jessica, incomplete images of myself, two men and a woman who represent the bracketed spectrum of an uncertain future. Soon I'll have been on the list nine months. Already I've endured two false alarms, one that nearly killed me. Since the second event I have felt myself quietly going mad as my physical and psychological limits are relentlessly challenged. I can barely walk about the house, my weight has ballooned from one hundred eighty-five pounds to two hundred twelve as a result of the water retention. As I lie back and witness the swelling of my legs and ankles, I grow acutely depressed, as though my existence is locked in a state of suspended animation, a state I am helpless to alter. Since mere breathing has become difficult, I decided to call Dr. Campbell yesterday. He told me that it's time, that I am now too ill to wait at home. Tomorrow I am to return to the hospital where I will be placed on heavy doses of Dobutamine until a donor heart is found. In preparation for the event Richard has arranged for a sofer, a holy scribe, to inscribe parchment, known as a mezuzah, from the Torah. He wants to ensure that my home is properly prepared in a kosher fashion before the transplant so that God might be with me.

The window stands vast and blank. The living room takes on the air of a tomb, a wintery sarcophagus, somnolent gurgles rise out of the hot water pipes throughout the house. I take up Elie Wiesel's *Night:* ". . . as of a Lazarus risen from the dead, yet still a prisoner within the grim confines where he had strayed, stumbling among the shameful corpses."

The sky thickens with snow, my mind fades into a gray whiteness, into a calm underworld. I feel my mind sleeping, intense, dreamless.

A moment later brightness fills the crimson panorama beneath the eyelids. I hear the soft patter of small feet descending the staircase, Abbe stirring beneath the heavy bedding. My mind awakens with the household. Looking at the wall clock I see I managed two hours of sleep, a rare achievement anymore.

Abbe glides into the kitchen, puts on a pot of coffee, and together we get my things for my final stay at the hospital. There is little talk. Small displays of affection keep the progress civilized. The sooner I get on the plane the better. I have been impossible lately, volatile and agitated, the anxiety having infected my demeanor.

At the airport a turboprop squats at the near end of the runway as it idles, the incandescent dorsal light flashing through the fog. Abbe and I move through the line at the ticket counter, then head for the single-room concourse. We gravely stare at one another for a moment, then wrap ourselves in the other's arms. I feel a sudden rush of tears, the weight of sadness as I press my face to the softness of her hair.

"I'll see you the day after tomorrow," she says.

"This will all be a vague memory soon."

"The kids will miss you."

I tell her how I can't seem to shake the insecurities over checking into the hospital knowing this will be my last time.

"This heart I have will be in a beaker the next time I see this valley. Either that or I'll be dead."

"You'll see the valley again," she says, pulling me into her. "They won't just let you die."

A whale-shaped cloud bank moves in as the propellers of the turboprop stand poised to cut it to ribbons. Damp snow stands in crumbling piles around the perimeter of the runway, revealing the clean and wet concrete. I make a weak attempt at a plaintive smile, say a final goodbye, and head out the door between two yellow strips of paint leading to the hatch in the belly of the plane. The exertion is all I can summon. As the plane lifts, the valley floor quickly vanishes in a bottomless haze.

It occurs to me as I walk down the hall to admissions that hospitals never change. The same antiseptic smells broken by the odor of feces and urine, the same harsh fluorescence, the same bland cafeteria food, the same bureaucracy. But it's a familiar setting, one I've grown comfortable being a part of through the years, I suppose. My depression lifts once I'm relaxing in bed, the traveling done, the questions asked, papers signed, blood drawn. Within days the ward has magically transformed itself into a neighborhood. When feeling well I'm asked to see other patients waiting on various transplant lists. I lug the IV carriage behind me as I move about the ward to sit and visit. I suddenly feel useful while sharing stories of false alarms, fears of not finding a donor in time, feelings of fragility. A strong and immediate bond is always formed, a feeling of solidarity.

But as the days slowly pass with me on my back, I witness the growing crest of my belly as the heart fails a little more each day. The belly feeds on heart failure. When lying back there's the constant sensation that I'm drowning in my own body fluid, being immersed in water, like a wave breaking over my chest.

The same difficulties plague simple tasks, such as keeping an IV line in my arm without blowing a vein. My arms are wrapped to the elbow in massive bruises. Then there are the newcomers, doctors and nurses who at first don't see placing an IV line in a solid vein as a problem. Their cocky naiveté sparks quick anger. "Trust me, it won't work, so don't try," I warn with a threatening seriousness they clearly don't expect. So every five to seven days a central line is threaded into the subclavian vein at the base of my neck. The procedure is surgical and carries the risk of infection and puncturing of the lung. Though the puncture risk is minimal, something like one in one thousand, they perform it often enough that the peril soon becomes very real. Distant odds are magnified, the terror of possibility becomes imaginable.

The backdrop to all this is a baneful nervousness as to whether or not I am to get a heart this very day, this very hour. There is absolutely no telling. I have to accept loss of control while facing impending death, which creates a fine edge of anxiety. The breadth of my faith is dictated by pendulous mood swings, which, in turn, are dictated by my current state of health. Good health translates into more time to find a donor organ. At these times I want to surround myself with friends, become swallowed by raucous voices. I convince myself I am to get a strong young heart. Health breeds time and time breeds confidence. But this very confidence is consistently leavened by hopelessness, feelings of complete despair, anger no one can relate to. I become acutely aware I am alone in this dilapidated body, and the only person who can undergo this transplant, or this death, is me. I stare into the darkness and the darkness stares back. The cosmos appears, after all, to be an infinitely dark and lonely place.

During these times all I want is to be left alone, to curl into myself, retreat into an autistic world and tend to my injured psyche, like a wounded animal crawling off to die. My chronic active disease devolves into chronic active self-absorption. I need a webby balm to heal myself, having fooled myself into believing I can do it alone. Self-absorption, I faintly suspect, could prove as lethal as IHSS. Intellectually I know this to be the case, though it's emotionally irresistible.

Then comes nightfall when I'm visited by dreams, convoluted nightmares populated with vaguely familiar faces. Fatal accidents occur, a car glides across the mountain road glazed with snow, then rotates through the air in slow circles as it floats down a ravine between powdered fir and aspen trees, coming to an abrupt halt against an outcropping of blue granite. The driver dies of a clean head wound, the back of his skull erupts, the neck breaks, severing the nervous system, fine vermilion capillaries bleed onto an intricately shattered windshield, and I awake with a shudder. I'm chilled with sweat, glaringly awake and cold. Reaching down I find I've worked the covers down to my ankles in a fit of nightmare.

A young person is going to die, I think to myself. That's why I am here, I am counting on it, staking my life on its occurrence. A young person with nothing physically wrong with them, a young person for whom I profess not to have any feelings of guilt. My first impulse is to rationalize it into a matter of fate. This unforeseeable death has nothing to do with Robert Pensack needing a heart: his death will occur whether I need a heart or not. It has been predetermined by an inscrutable god.

I pause, close my eyes against the darkness.

Small voices leak through the broad wooden door. I strain to listen, a tactic to sidetrack the mind. Night passes, the soft tumblers of thought continue their invisible work. Then it dawns on me, rising up from a recessed portion of the brain, like a silhouette approaching through fog. I am feeling guilt after all. That I am going through this thought process is evidence of guilt, small traces haunting my dreams.

To some this may seem obvious. Of course it's guilt; I benefit as a result of another's misfortune. Without this death, my life ends. I want this death to occur, I look forward to it happening. But these are thoughts the mind hides from itself, allowing them to smolder like a fire in the pantry with no chimney. But the smoke escapes, and it does so in dreams. Thus, thoughts of guilt are at once obvious and obscure.

But ultimately these thoughts are flawed: I do not look forward to this death, and I do wish it were avoidable. What I look forward to is a new heart, new life. That's all.

So the night passes, laden with moral dilemma, with the splitting of dialectical hairs.

32

A young nurse leans against the doorjamb with a blood pressure cuff draped over her wrist. She stares down, her eyes fixed on the other side of a brown clipboard, collecting data on the peculiar workings of my body. She introduces herself as Laura, my nurse for the next eleven hours, then approaches the bed and sits on the edge. I notice she's pretty in a matronly sort of way. I watch her as she scans my charts without speaking, her breath wheezing through her upturned nose. Already I feel the onset of maternal attachment. She softly clucks her tongue as she reads in silence. Then, with delicate surprise, she says, "So, you've been on the transplant list for a while."

"Nine months now."

"I was with Mr. Debey the night he got his heart."

I struggle to sit up. "You were there?"

"Oh yes. He hooted and hollered like he'd scored a touchdown." She gazes toward the window, her eyes taking in the distance. "It was quite a celebration that night." She brings her eyes back to the clipboard and returns to the business at hand. The ward is a busy place today.

But my interest is piqued, I want to know the circumstances, how it occurred, who called, everything.

"When did he get the call?" My voice is warbled with excitement.

"Oh, let's see . . ." She lazily brings a finger to her chin. "It was in the evening. Late in the evening. About ten or eleven, I'd say."

"And who called? Who was the first person to tell you they had a heart for Mr. Debey?"

"I believe it was Dr. Lindenfeld, actually."

"JoAnn Lindenfeld, Dr. Lindenfeld?"

"Yes, that's right. Dr. Lindenfeld." She nods, fixing her eyes on the charts.

But I've only just begun. I come at Laura with a battery of questions concerning every aspect of that night. I want to know it all, to master it, to understand what manifested the call, uncover the invisible structure of organ appropriation. Soon she becomes visibly weary of the interrogation as I begin asking questions twice. I never tire of hearing the same story over and over, and ask revised versions of the same questions in an attempt to surround the event, reveal its depth and breadth.

Eventually she takes my arm and wraps it in a Velcro cuff and begins thrusting air into the pocket with short quick contractions of her small fist. I continue the probe, oblivious to the tourniquet of air about my bicep. She answers in monotone, looking down at her wristwatch as air escapes in a steady hiss. Then she abruptly stands and asks if that will be all. I nod and say of course. Before escaping out the door, she adds the new numbers to the long columns as a final act.

Later that afternoon I rummage through my wallet, pulling out memorabilia from the outside world: directions on a napkin, business cards, phone numbers. Looking at the dark creases in the leather, I think of the places it's been with me, riding on my hip like a tattoo, an instrument of daily life. On a folded square of a legal sheet I find Jimmy's number, the guy who contracted the virus that destroyed his heart while stationed in the Persian Gulf.

I pound out the numbers while silently rehearsing the questions I want to ask concerning the events leading up to the call. Even for this man, I am thinking, I feel the pang of jealousy. He has a new young heart, and I don't.

We talk about current matters first, his recovery, my wait, the importance of emotional stamina. Jimmy speaks excitedly, optimistically, about the rapture he feels simply being alive. He makes discreet references to his faith, gentle probes into the state of my faith. I ask my questions concerning the night of his call and he gives me a few details, and speaks of the will of God, Faith, Hope, giving away little concrete information about the actual historical circumstances. Toward the end of the conversation he says he'll be praying for me, and offers a verse from the book of Matthew, a passage that helped him get through the ordeal.

"I'll look it up," I say. "But one last thing, Jimmy. What was the recovery like, those first couple of weeks? Was it incredibly tough?"

He pauses, then says, "Bob, it's a war. You've got to be *an animal.*"

"I understand."

I lie back, looking up at the familiar pattern in the ceiling tiles for several minutes. When Laura comes in, I ask her if there's a Bible on the ward, one with a New Testament. She says she'll look around, and fifteen minutes later returns with hands in the air. "There's not a Bible on the ward. Not a one."

"Imagine that." Morbid laughter rises from deep within. Here we are, a ward of the most chronically ill people in the state, and there's not a Bible to be found. Laura doesn't appear to appreciate the irony and leaves, looking a little disappointed, a little concerned. The laughter keeps coming for some time after she has left, but eventually gives way to a kind of jealousy of those capable of genuine religious faith. It must be easier. It has to be. Whether solace comes from religious myth taken literally, alcohol or misplaced trust in medical science, they are all more comforting than what the agnostic allows himself: nervous superstition, hope based strictly on arithmetic.

That night old friends come by. Jake is an emergency room physician. His girlfriend Michelle is with him now as they stand in the doorway, quietly greeting me without words, only concerned meager smiles as they approach the bed. Michelle shrugs off her coat and hugs my head and shoulders in one smooth motion, and asks how I am holding up.

"Not too well, actually," I say, inhaling the sharp perfume of her blond hair. When she releases me, Jake surrounds me in his long arms. There is a moment of easy silence.

"So Abbe's in Steamboat?" Jake asks.

"She's up there taking care of the children until this happens."

We talk about mutual friends, Jake's practice, what I hope to do after the transplant, assuming there will be a transplant, and that it will be successful, that the body won't reject the heart, that I will be sane . . .

"I bought you something that might help," Jake says. He reaches deep into his leather coat pocket and produces a handful of cassette tapes held together by a blue rubber band. "They're relaxation tapes, something to listen to before they put you under."

"With subliminal messages?" I ask.

"Propaganda to sleep by."

I think of Jimmy, the book of Matthew, then say thanks and set the tapes on the windowsill next to a stack of unread magazines. Trying not to appear ungracious, I tell Jake relaxation tapes are not my thing. This heart transplant to me is WAR. I point out my Marine-like crew cut, I grit my teeth and widen my eyes like a maniac.

Then the conversation settles for a while on Abbe, the kids, and feelings I have of being misunderstood. I tell them how the frustration of waiting for this heart threatens my marriage. Jake's voice is calm and soothing. My mind dwells as he subtly promotes gravitation toward ambiguous faith. Faith. Then Laura steps into our company, modest, careful of being intrusive, her hands clasped before her like those of a maître d'. My eyes arc, dazed with thought, across the room.

"Sorry, Bob," she says, extending her neck. "There's a call for you at the nurses' station."

"Who is it, Laura?"

"It's Dr. Lindenfeld."

I magically hop up as though never ill. I try to speak: "It's JoAnn Lindenfeld. It's a heart. They've got a heart for me . . ."

I hobble through the doorway and head directly for the counter where another nurse holds a phone in her hand like a torch, her eyes smiling, her lips bitten and pale. This is it, I whisper, this is it. I feel an electric tingle from the summit to the base of my spine. I read her every gesture as I approach: the drawn line of her eyes, the thin line of her mouth, the lens of the eyes glassy with mild tears. Without a word she thrusts the phone onto my shoulder below the ear.

". . . Bob . . . This is what we've been waiting for. We've got a very large heart from a very large young man. But it's in Texas . . ."

"A heart . . ."

". . . We think this is it, Bob. It's big and it's young . . ."

"Big and young."

"But it's in Corpus Christi. Dave Campbell is on his way down now to harvest."

33

The voice, JoAnn's voice, vanishes with a click. Yet I hold the receiver to my ear for an appreciable time, intensely reluctant to be far from it, afraid to be out of touch. Slowly, half-consciously, the receiver slides from my shoulder onto my breast, and I begin to cry, soft and easy at first, then uncontrollably in hard unrestrained bursts.

Laura makes her way around the counter, and I reach out to pull her into me. I hardly know this woman, she is but a vague acquaintance in the neighborhood of the ward. Yet she is now close and uninhibited, graciously taking me into her body, intuiting my need for human touch, community. The crying penetrates beyond expressions of happiness, relief, release from pain, even hope of salvation. The tears intensify just when decorum suggests it's time to pull myself together. The breakdown is complete; I sense a phenomenon beyond my control at work, something rooted in the psyche that has bled into my skin like an indelible dye.

All the while Laura keeps hold of me, though she too is a little startled by the thoroughness of the collapse. There's a new clarity in my mind as to the depth of the pain I've lived with. I see now, as my body convulses apart, the intensity of feeling my defenses have protected me from.

"Do you want to call your wife, Bob?"

I raise my chin from her shoulder, finally feeling the tears begin to ebb.

"I don't think I can."

"Would you like me to?"

I nod yes like a small boy and release her, carefully loosening my arms about her neck as if easing them away. My body feels weak now, thoroughly drained of energy. If I spoke with Abbe I'm afraid I'd break down all over again, feel the sudden inexorable rush of tears and cry till there was nothing but a puddle left. I simply can't speak to Abbe, I tell myself, for fear I'll realize I'm dreaming. The person I want to talk to, the only person I *can* talk to, is my father. I am a child now and need my parent.

I tell Laura and she whispers her understanding. She then takes me by the shoulders and gently steers me toward my room with an arm across my back. I look up to see Jake and Michelle standing just outside the doorway, smiling as I approach. Again, I am taken into arms, smothered by human warmth.

"It's happening," I say, my face compressed against their bodies, voice muted.

"What can we do?" Jake asks.

"Nothing."

I release myself and head into the room. I walk to the edge of the bed, sit down and stare at the phone on the night table, considering in the relative silence who should receive the news first. If I call Abbe, I'll break down again. I know this. And I'll wear myself out. Moreover, I may jinx the new heart; they might discover a flaw, call it off for reasons all their own. If I tell the most important person to me in the world, it will be called off. If I call Richard I suspect I will be overwhelmed with dogma and prayers. At the moment I need simple love and empathy. Not wanting to take any chances, rational or otherwise, I decisively take up the phone with a jerk and press the small gray buttons to my father's home in New Jersey.

His wife, Joan, answers, and I excitedly tell her I need to talk to them both on the phone.

"Is something wrong?" she asks.

"Something's very right."

I hear her call him, and eventually his grim concerned voice says my name.

"They've got a heart for me, Dad. It's big and young and in Texas. You need to book the first flight out in the morning."

Both voices come at me at once, garbled and excited. I hear Dad getting discombobulated in his familiar concerned manner.

"Are they sure this time?" he asks with the first break of silence.

"Dad, they're never sure."

"Well, why don't you call just before you go down to the OR, before I book our flight?"

"Dad. This is going to happen. This is the last time you will hear my voice before I wake up in the ICU."

He mumbles his understanding, his voice reluctant, his faceless voice conveying trepidation for fear of mishap. We exchange our love, pause, then I reiterate my boundless optimism. He says he'll see me when I wake up. With that I slowly lower the phone into the cradle. I sit on the edge of the bed in silence for some time, then turn to see Jake and Michelle standing quietly together, at once trying to stay out of the way and be at my disposal. Their matching ineffable expressions say it all. Disbelief, awe, the hand of harmonic convergence. A simple visit, and now this. Suddenly Laura scurries through the door talking rapidly.

"I called Abbe and she said she'll be on the next flight out of Steamboat which arrives here at 9:05 P.M." Her efficiency is intended to put me at ease, and it does. Jake and Michelle promptly offer to pick her up.

"Everything seems to be falling into place," I say.

"It's your show, Bob," Laura says.

Soon the room is inundated with doctors and nurses with a volley of questions. Someone places the familiar forms on my belly that release them from responsibility, another draws my blood into a long plastic cylinder. That there is no other known course of action, that this is a last-resort measure is made clear to me in the familiar stilted language stated in the last false alarm. This is heroic medicine, it is charged with risk. The pain I will feel upon awakening will continue for weeks; it will be both intense and long-lasting. I will be terrified, wonder if it was ever worth it. I may feel the surgeons have robbed me of my personality, having taken away my heart, the center of my being. Of course they don't explain all of this; it is mostly a mental rehearsal I am going through. I know what to expect and I expect the very best, though even the best-case scenario is perilous. I am going through with this. I am going to ease through it. Tonight I am a lucky man. There is a sense of synchronicity about the night that hasn't shown itself until now. I will never die. I think of the second false alarm, a weak heart bruised by a heater door exploding off its hinges. Luck glitters in the night like small jewels, like stars. Its presence is palpable like the ghost of a loved one haunting the ward.

Then the ringing of the phone pierces the skein of thought. I reluctantly pick it up and hear Richard's sharp urgent voice telling me he heard the news through Dad.

"That's right. But it's still in Texas," I say.

"*Baruch Hashem.* I want to point out the significance of this day on the Hebrew calendar," he begins before I interrupt him.

"Richard, I have to go," I say. "I love you very much, but there's a lot going on right now."

"I'll be praying for you, Bob." And we hang up.

After a long quiet pause I see Jake whisper to Michelle, then quietly announce they'd better be going to the airport. It's 8:45 P.M., time has been compressed beyond recognition.

Within what seems but a handful of seconds, Abbe comes bustling through the doorway, her arms parted. The plane was late, she explains, her face worried, hopeful, apologetic.

"I never would have known," I say. "Everything's happening so fast." We hug each other long and hard knowing this will be one of the last. "It's happening tonight, Ab. I'm due in the OR at 11:00."

"The heart's in Texas?" she asks.

"I'll talk like Ross Perot next week."

"You'll sit around all day hatching conspiracy theories."

"It's that simple. I'm Ross and you're the boss."

I'm feeling giddy now, full of the thrilling knowledge that I'm going to be around awhile. It's no longer hope, but knowledge. I am way ahead of myself. As time progresses, the circle of doctors and nurses tightens around me, a flurry of voices occasionally interrupted by a word of warning before a needle slides into my forearm. Old friends from medical school arrive making their way through the crowd to wish luck, a successful surgery. The energy invigorates, makes me manic. I want to stand and move about to vent the electricity, but the preliminaries won't be completed until it's time to go. Eventually Mike Grosso, a thoracic surgeon on the transplant team, parts the crowd and places his fists on his hips and smiles.

"It's a go. I just talked with Dave. He's in Corpus Christi right now and he says it looks great."

My head bobs. I feel its lightness. I want to ask him to repeat the words only to hear them again. *It's a go.*

"Did you hear that, Ab?" I whisper.

"We're on a stopwatch now. We need to see you down in the OR by 11:00. See you down there." And he vanishes.

I nod. No fear. None whatsoever. My heart is on its way. Corpus Christi, blood of my blood, flesh of my flesh, memory of my memory.

Within minutes JoAnn Lindenfeld appears at the foot of the bed. She is smiling wide, the first time I've ever seen joy in her eyes. She bears good news.

"I just received a FAX of the EKGs. They look excellent."

"I knew they would," I say. She floats her small cool palm into mine. "Can I give you a kiss, JoAnn?" I ask.

"Of course you can." And I do.

Soon Mike reappears and announces that it's time to leave. Behind him a male nurse navigates a wheelchair through the crowd to the side of the bed, and I climb into its cold vinyl lap. Abbe propels the chair down the hall with doctors, nurses and friends in our wake. As we stroll into the elevator an anesthesiologist pulls a clear oxygen mask over my face. The doors wheeze open, we zigzag through the corridors, Abbe pets my head as we approach the OR. There is no fear, no foreboding. The windowless doors grow within the scope of vision as we slowly surge on, voices chat with eerie nervousness, I hear myself speak, make jokes. The doors magically part, Abbe and I exchange our final kiss. I tell her everything will be fine, and tell myself I'll never die.

Beyond the door is the sudden familiar sterile landscape, the green uniforms of pale zombies who work through the night, who go for days without sleep. It is a windowless environment with the secure air of a cellar or tomb, where lights burn over reposed bodies of the near-dead as though lit by amphetamines. A sleepless chamber. They roll me into the very room where I witnessed Dr. Starzl perform a liver transplant on a two-and-a-half-year-old girl twenty years ago. A good omen; the mind reels.

I'm wheeled in beside the operating table where I stand, carefully lifting my arms bristling with IV wires, then hoist myself onto its cold upholstery. Now I too lie reposed. I look up into the huge disk of harsh surgical light, my arms splayed out crosslike, feeling the cool vinyl warm against the small of my back. The voices of friends surround me along with the hurried clatter of preparation. Two hands descend about my temples with the faceless voice of Jon Berman, an old friend, an anesthesiologist, saying, It's time for your glasses, Bobby, and their weight is gone, replaced by grainy vision. There are now only voices against a backdrop of clatter. Here I am, looking into brightness. Another mask is brought over my face, I am told to count backward, I am told nightie-night, Bobby. The deeper I spin. Again I tell myself I will never die.

RAISING LAZARUS

34

Plastic tape covers both eyes, like coins in the eyes of the dead. All hair is shaved from Adam's apple to groin, exposing the naked dome of my belly. Ancient scars are revealed, tissue toughened and darkened through the process of healing. The skin is then painted in betadine, a disinfectant the color of molten gold when dried to flesh.

Mike Grosso stands over my body wearing a headlamp and Woody Allen glasses that brighten and magnify what lies before his scalpel. He glances every now and then at the wall clock so that his surgery and the arrival of the absent heart will be choreographed as one motion, not arriving too early or late. My body temperature will be lowered to 80 degrees Fahrenheit, my blood oxygenated by a machine acting as heart and lungs for several hours. So Mike stands idle till the clock advances to the point that the dissection of my heart will coordinate with the arrival of its replacement from Corpus Christi. My sternum is superimposed onto the grid of his mind's eye, and a measurement made just below the valley of the glottis. Eventually he makes the initial cut with the confidence bred by the acuity required of heart surgeons.

I'm cutting, he announces to no one in particular. Just a vague bulletin of where he's at relative to the approaching heart. It is 12:18 in the morning.

The scalpel moves along the old scar like a knife over the seam of a peach, exposing small pouches of fat cells and seventeen-year-old baling wire. Once the incision is complete, Fred Grover, a pulmonary surgeon experienced in lung transplantation, nonchalantly wanders in and surveys the progress. His surgical gloves are pristine, unlike Mike's, which are now smudged crimson. Fred quietly looks on as Mike lifts the old scar tissue from the center of my chest like a strip of brain coral. The baling wire is now in full view. Together they untwist the steel filaments with pliers, then gently tug them from the healed bone.

A surgical nurse stands at the side of each surgeon, while an anesthesiologist hovers above my head, partially separated from view by a stunted curtain. The saw comes to life in Mike's hand, quietly humming with precision. He begins at the summit of the sternum then slowly works the small whirring blade down to six inches above the navel. He's very easy with the saw, not wanting to cut too deeply, yet enough so as to separate what is one broad bone protecting the most vital organs. Once he thinks he's finished, he peers into the thin crevice flooded with lamplight to see if the bone is entirely separated. Finding small sections where he hasn't cut deeply enough, he lowers the scalpel into the kerf and cuts through the thin shards. By pressing a button on the scalpel handle, he can either cut or burn through flesh, cauterizing the incision. When burning, a feather of yellow smoke spirals over the cautery, filling the air with the unforgettable odor of scalded flesh.

Once bound with steel, now unbound. The sternum is in two, the halves floating upon the lungs as on clouds. Small retractors—aluminum rakelike instruments—are placed between the two halves, then Mike and Fred gently tug them apart from opposite sides of the table. The bone is rigid and thick; they pull with most of their strength, then once a small chasm is formed, an aluminum spreader is set between the halves and the sternum pried apart. My insides glisten within the scarlet gap, the heart secretly quivers fast and alive.

Fred now looks on, subtly commenting on where to cut and where to burn away the adhesions and tissue cradling the heart. The chasm is gently widened simultaneously: a little is cut, the spreader gapes, revealing the slow tired thrusts of a sick organ. The tissue responds to the touch of the knife, shyly shrinking from contact beneath a small pillar of yellow smoke as if the flesh itself were sentient, capable of memory and desire. Soon the heart is wholly revealed.

Well, by golly, progress, Fred says.

Mike glances over his shoulder to the wall clock and states the time, 1:03 A.M. He doesn't want to work too far ahead, but it's time to start considering bypass. The machine squats beside the operating table with two nurses sitting next to it on short stools, the ensemble ready and waiting to act as heart and lungs until the new pump belongs to my body and is capable of sustaining life.

Suddenly the stereo comes alive with Beethoven's Fifth. Mike and Fred continue to work, further revealing the cradle of the heart until the aorta, vena cava and pulmonary artery and veins are in full view. The body retreats from the heart as the knife warns it away.

Mike wags his head in disbelief as he sinks his hand into the chest cavity around the heart to feel its slow stiff labor. He suddenly senses an irregular beat and removes his hand, allowing it to recover. Above my head a row of monitors confirms what he felt in his palm. The blood pressures drop slightly, the rhythm stumbles. That's the sickest-looking right atrium I've ever seen, Mike says, pointing to the purple striations in the muscle.

Looks like your typical transplant heart to me, Fred says.

Clear plastic tubes from the heart-lung machine are brought

up to the chest, then small rubber ties are looped about the vena cava. The small nooses are left loose until every aspect of bypass is ready, then they are constricted, inhibiting blood flow. At that point the blood is rerouted through the tubes to the bypass machine, where it is enriched with oxygen and returned to the body at the trunk of the aorta.

Someone asks when Dave is expected to arrive; Fred answers, Anytime now. Meanwhile, he and Mike begin the actual dissection. It convulses, nearly to a halt, a few seconds after the clamping of arteries and veins commences. At 1:59 A.M. the right side of the heart is entirely bypassed, the chambers fibrillate every now and then, but they are generally flaccid and still. They will never beat again.

Fred watches on as Mike severs the vena cava. At 2:05 they're ready to bypass the left side of the heart. Mike taps air bubbles out of the plastic tubes with clamps, as they pose the threat of stroke. Heparin, an anticoagulant, is administered intravenously to keep the blood from clotting upon entering the oxygen-rich catacombs of the heart-lung machine. This of course raises the risk of bleeding, but there is no alternative. Blood tends to clot when oxygenated artificially, so it is anticoagulated.

At 2:06 A.M. the swinging doors of the OR flop open, and in slides a maroon Igloo picnic cooler across the polished concrete floor. Heart's here, the nurse at Mike's side announces. Dave remains outside. A few minutes later, he strides in to view my status, then leaves, pleased that the process has been coordinated within a few minutes of his arrival. The heart is nearly ready to be lifted out and the new one brought to bear. Presently it lies dormant, chilled and quieted with ice and potassium, poised to function again at the bidding of a gentle flicker of electricity.

The anesthesiologist asks Dave the cause of death.

Farming accident, he says, gazing over Fred's shoulder. I see you're almost ready for me.

We're almost there, Fred replies.

Dave walks to the cooler, opens the lid and carefully lifts the fresh young heart up to the light with both hands to check for contusions and blemishes. The coronary arteries gleam in the lamplight. A very large, very young human heart. Meanwhile, Fred and Mike lift my dissected heart from my chest, leaving an incomprehensible cavity.

Within minutes Mike announces they're ready. Dave approaches the table with the heart in his hands, inspecting it one last time, then lays it into the chest. Without a heart I resemble a dugout canoe, I may later imagine.

Now the sewing commences. My old right atrium is left partially intact so that only one large incision need be made instead of two in order to accommodate the superior and inferior vena cava. The pulmonary artery and my original left atrial cuff is then sewn to the new heart, and finally the aorta. The work isn't especially delicate. Unlike a liver transplant, this is the connecting of pipelike arteries and veins. So progress is quick, but then it has to be. Judging by the clock, Mike estimates the heart will have been stopped for six and a half hours by the time they're ready for electricity. Generally they like to stay under four. Though surgeons have successfully transplanted hearts that have been stopped for as long as eight hours, they've also had difficulty restarting hearts stopped for only two. A messy science. This heart from Corpus Christi is at the margins of acceptable risk.

By 3:40 A.M. the sewing is nearly complete. The nooses are loosened, the heart filled with blood, residual air is then gently eased from the chambers. The circulatory system is complete, though the new heart lies static while the heart-lung machine feeds the blood to the body. For some time now the heart has been warmed slowly in preparation for its first movements. At 3:46 A.M. small electric paddles are brought to the chest. Mike carefully places one against the left atrium, the other upon the right ventricle. He gives the word to release electricity, and the organ quivers upon its arrival. The heart belongs to me now.

Again. And the atrium fibrillates a little.

Again.

More atrial fibrillation, but it fades quickly, and the heart's movement conforms to a beating pattern. The thrusting motion is unmistakable, the familiar efficient coordination of a heart pumping blood as this one has for twenty years. But the motion remains equivocal and not entirely deliberate in nature, as though the organ were relearning what it had forgotten while out of a body. Now it lies in me, dazed and confused.

The blood the heart moves is merely supplemental to that the heart-lung machine pumps, which is the way it will be until the new heart is strong enough to sustain life on its own. Above my head the row of monitors measures my every body function, including several blood pressures. Not until the pressures are much higher will it be safe to come off bypass. So far they are frighteningly low, the heart barely pumping. The room grows quiet, the mood palpably dour as the pressures fail to rise as expected. Drugs that stimulate the heart muscle are administered intravenously, thereby increasing the pressures artificially. This works to a limited extent.

That's a pretty good-sized heart, Dave says, observing the dramatic thrashing motion. In comparison to the old one, the donor heart is enormous, its movement emphatic, but inefficient.

I just wish it would move more blood, Mike says.

Hopefully it will soon, Dave replies. He then asks Fred if he needs a break, and Fred says he'll be back in a few minutes. Before vanishing through the swinging doors he speaks with one of the cardiac nurses in a hushed voice. After their short conversation she heads to the phone and says plaintively, We need more blood products. We've got a bleeder down here. Then she carefully sets the receiver down, sits beside the other cardiac nurse and stares ahead blankly. This one's in deep shit. The other nods in agreement, her naked arms wrapped tight about her waist against the chill. His pressures really haven't gone up in the last hour, she says.

Meanwhile new heart-stimulant drugs are discussed, along with means of controlling the bleeding that is slowly but implacably getting worse. Every now and then the chortling sound of suction fills the room. The longer I'm on the machine the more heparin I require; hence the blood doesn't clot. Yet I can't come off bypass until the pressures rise. So it all comes down to questions of the heart: will it get stronger—and soon? Situations like this are renowned for gaining a corrosive momentum of their own, spinning out of control with sheer mindless centrifugal force. Presently the bleeding is relatively minor and controllable, but considering its poor performance so far, and the shallow rate of improvement, danger is clear and present.

Mike and Dave work on with steady aplomb, trying various drugs, one at a time, to stimulate cardiac output. The results are swiftly gauged, the improvement or lack of improvement assessed, new tactics imagined and discussed. By 6:00 A.M. I'm still on bypass, though every now and then they try to take me off only to watch the pressures plummet. But gradually, imperceptibly and painstakingly the pressures do rise, though not enough to keep me alive. And the bleeding worsens. The gurgle of suction is now constant.

As alternatives are discussed, the use of a balloon pump to assist the heart comes up. The pump would enter the femoral artery in the groin, and help raise my blood pressure by acting as a sort of auxiliary. It is an impromptu measure. The decision of whether or not to use it comes down to the question of whether or not it will get me off bypass sooner. The conventional wisdom is that it can't help much. But it can't hurt either. The potential for bleeding, subtle brain damage and stroke is lessened, so the decision to go with it is made. Within minutes the incision is deftly executed into my right femoral artery, and the device inserted.

Meanwhile, four stories above my sleeping body, above the mounting tension of the siege, my wife opens her eyes in the predawn darkness to the thin crest of flaxen light fading to violet. For a brief moment she doesn't know where she is until recognizing the familiar slats of the Venetian blinds. Then it all comes rushing back in her vague state between dream and consciousness. She now knows where she is, why she's here, and a smile forms as she nuzzles her cheek into the bedding. Her thoughts are suddenly flooded with the memory of the phone call, the confidence, the bravado, the promise of new life. She keeps her eyes open for a moment to take in the warm sensation of luck's return to our lives, together with the tactile warmth of the hospital bed, and the new light mounting the horizon. After briefly wondering what it was that woke her, she slips back into quiet sleep.

35

By 6:30 A.M. the bypass machine is rolled away. My heart together with the balloon pump is keeping my blood pressure adequate—the bleeding, however, is now out of hand. When Mike takes a break he stops at the phone on his way, his voice grim and confidential. It doesn't get any worse than this, he explains over the phone. We'll need plenty more blood products down here. Already I've taken fifty units; blood-soaked rags fill a half-dozen clear plastic bags surrounding the operating table. It's remarkable how problems replace themselves instead of simply going away once solved.

The work is tedious and seemingly pointless. Having been bypassed for more than four hours, the blood has absorbed an enormous amount of heparin. In spite of efforts at controlling the bleeding, it simply grows worse in randomness. At the same time the heart has swelled with the accumulation of stress like a gigantically inflamed tonsil. Though it appears vigorous and healthy as it thrashes about in the cavity, no one is entirely certain whether this heart is any good. And another ambush lies in wait. For the moment it is left unsaid in lieu of more urgent problems at hand, but the question of how to close my chest around such a grossly swollen heart has silently presented itself.

Since trouble arose the radio has changed in format from classical to rock and roll, and steadily grown louder. The music is white noise, a blank point of reference that focuses the sleepless mind. The surgeons have been working for nearly ten hours, and Dave longer still, having been to the southern tip of Texas to harvest the heart, and flown back. And who's to say how long any of them had worked before they received the call? These things are always unexpected. The team seems to thrive on sleep deprivation, like a tribe of nocturnal beings driven by fear of nightmare. Now Dave returns to the table after a brief rest in the lounge, and says as he approaches the table, Okay, Bob, it's just you and me. He has unmistakable presence at the table. His feet and shoulders bob in constant rhythm as though he were shadow-boxing over the patient, ducking and weaving, working quickly through long intense bouts.

As he and Fred focus on the bleeding, the pressures slowly rise. By 10:20 A.M. the heart's working just as well with the balloon pump as without. And the anesthesiologist is more hopeful too since he has begun to administer fewer drugs to stimulate cardiac output. But this is the good news. Above me on the TV monitor the laborious thrusts of the enormous organ fill the screen.

The surgeons continue to rotate through the late morning hours and eventually abate the bleeding after sixty units of blood. The pressures are now up, the heart strong and relatively compliant. Then at 11:20 A.M. Mike and Dave try to close for the first time. Baling wire is woven into the tiny drill holes, the silver filaments fan across my chest like an arc of porcupine quills. As the two halves of the sternum are eased together, the heart silently retreats from view. Only an inch-wide fissure now remains. But as they bring the bones together the monitors show what has been feared all along. The pressures suddenly plummet as the heart is compressed, unable to fill completely. They immediately part the sternum and the heart recovers. This is dire. My immune system is suppressed and must stay so, leaving me wide-open to infection if they can't close right away. It could take several days in the ICU with my chest gaping until the swelling goes down. Mike and Dave try again to close only to discover the same result. This doesn't look good, Mike says. We might have to wait until the swelling goes down.

All the while Jon Berman has been quietly observing, his eyes somber above the mask. He abruptly steps out the swinging doors with his head down, sullen and meditative. He has been in and out of the OR through the night tracking my status. Just outside the room where I lie, Abbe sits in a metal folding chair next to a phone, legs crossed at the ankles, her small hands clenched around the leather strap of a handbag. An hour ago she called the ICU to see if I'd arrived, assuming the surgery was certainly over by now. No one had contacted and informed her of the outcome as she'd expected. No word since she last held my head in her hands and we kissed. Our life's about to change, I had said. After ten hours of silence she called the ICU, and the nurse on duty said they hadn't seen me, that she understood they were having some trouble downstairs. Abbe suddenly felt shocky, her skin hot and damp all over. Oh, she said into the receiver, her voice harsh and flat, not believing what the nurse had just told her. She slapped the phone down without another word then scurried out the door to the elevator, silently wondering what all the confusion could be about as she descended in the center of the quiet crowded vestibule. It couldn't possibly be Bob the nurse was speaking of. Absolutely not. This hospital is sometimes too big for its own good, she thought to herself. All this needless anxiety caused by misinformation.

By the time she was approaching the familiar hallway to the OR she felt better about the whole business. All looked normal as it should. No hints of emergency. She would walk through the doors, ask the receptionist where Bob was, and simply go there. The best doctors and surgeons in the nation and nobody knows what anyone else is doing, she mumbled as she strode through the broad swinging doors. When the setting of relaxed surgeons and doctors presented itself, she was further put at ease. Immediately she headed for the reception desk where the attending nurse told her in no uncertain terms that she didn't know, that she couldn't help her. So she went directly to the metal folding chair beneath the phone where she would calmly wait until someone came along whom she knew and could tell her where the hell Bob was and how he was doing. Her wait was short. She now sees Jon Berman walking toward her, his dark eyes gloomy, his arms lifted behind his head to untie his mask. They see each other at precisely the same moment. She stands and calls his name. He pauses then walks right up to her and begins to speak, slowly, obviously choosing his words with care, his voice steady but weary.

They've been having trouble with the new heart, Abbe. Bob's not doing so well. They may not be able to close today.

She gazes into the mouth from which the words came. No way . . . The voice is accusatory. She doesn't believe what she just heard. Jon glances away, then returns his eyes to hers. Her hands tighten into small fists, she wants to pound on his chest until he tells her something different. The desire is irresistible, almost reflex in nature. She suddenly feels a peculiar sensation, a dizzy wave of disorientation, dislocation from her environment as though she has slipped out of her body. She hears Jon say her name and make an explanation, picking up the muffled words "bleeding," "swelling," and "out of control," as though said in a large auditorium. She then hears her own voice chanting disbelief, anger. Jon absorbs it all. He tells her she should sit for a moment, gather her wits, but she defiantly refuses. Eventually she turns back toward the chair and sits. She stares dead ahead, her vision tunnel-like, the scope narrowed to what lies directly between her and the furthest end of the hallway. Peripheral objects gradually dim until there is but a small focus of light. She tries to speak, but unexpectedly—utterly unexpected to her—a hot burst of tears jet from her eyes. She inhales with a violent manic gasp and brings her small hands to her face.

After Fred relieves him for lunch, Mike Grosso morosely heads through the OR doors, and down the elevator to the cafeteria. Then, before joining the line, he slowly turns about and detours down a murky corridor that accesses the hospital utilities. The floor is concrete, the walls made up of bare pipes and wires. A constant hum broken by the muffled traffic of feet and equipment passing above fills the dank corridor. There is about it the atmosphere of a crypt or mummy chamber. He paces its length back and forth, moving along, head down, his mind turning in unison with the quick cadence of his short steps. The atmosphere alternately dampens and dries as he paces back and forth. Light condensation has collected on the concrete and pipes. Eventually he emerges from the half-light and consistent hum to the bustle of the cafeteria, the noise of plastic cutlery, hospital chatter and shoptalk.

He moves through the line lost in thought, then sits to eat alone, his eyes far away, lost on a wall. Colleagues pass unnoticed, a grateful patient greets him and is met with his dazed eyes and delayed look of recognition. How are you? he asks, not entirely able to shake the preoccupation. The patient, undaunted, goes on to explain in fine detail his present condition. Mike struggles to involve himself in the conversation, and does so for a while before they part. He then heads back to the elevator, back down the familiar fluorescent-lit halls. He quickly ties on a fresh mask, scrubs and pulls on a new pair of gloves, then approaches the table with his eyes on the row of monitors. He sees Dave and Fred have me wide-open again, but apparently Dave has come up with the potential solution of cutting away old adhesions, thereby making room for the swollen heart. And inexplicably the swelling has gone down some, though still not enough to close. There is a new confidence in the room. All three surgeons smile behind their masks.

Dave works fast in his athletic manner, as he excavates the chest cavity. It's past noon, and I've now been under anesthesia for more than twelve hours. The sheer time with the mind snowed on anesthesia, sunk into that small death called sleep, is now of primary concern. They need to be finishing up here as every minute on the table brings greater risk of anoxia. And they do so. By 12:30 P.M. they are ready to try closing again. Dave has swiftly and dramatically found what he thinks to be adequate space in his own mercurial fashion. Again they bring the two bones together and watch the effects of compression on the monitor above. The numbers remain steady as the bones slowly float together like the tectonic motion of continents and Mike and Dave glance back and forth between the monitor and wound. When the bones are but a half-inch apart they gaze up to see the numbers have held. Almost there, Mike mumbles. Almost there. As the bones meet, they again look up and nod at the numbers, steadfast on the screen. I am now whole. There is no time for congratulations, and the binding commences at once.

Just after 1:00 P.M. they begin stapling the wound, then take me off anesthesia altogether. Preparations begin for the quick trip in the elevator to the transplant ICU. Once I am stapled together, Jon Berman steps out of the OR to tell Abbe they've now got me closed, that at least I won't wake up with my hands tied down so that I don't dip them into my chest cavity. Though the news is good, the crisis survived for the moment, his voice remains grave. He doesn't candy-coat my condition, knowing the foolishness in spouting erroneous optimism. My situation is still dire. No one except Dave is optimistic. I am still in, as Jon says, kimchi. What he thinks but doesn't say is that even if I do get through the forest, if I don't die of rampant infection, if my kidneys do not die by poisoning, if I don't experience acute rejection, that I won't be Bob when I recover from the surgery. I was on a heart-lung machine nearly three hours longer than I should have been—nearly twice as long. That defining, immutable Self may have been altered, diminished. I very well could be little more than a talking monkey after this. But he restricts the conversation to immediate dangers, reassuring with reservations, guarding hints of confidence, and qualifying everything he says. He's more than willing to take the fall if all comes up roses. His experience, and it is vast, tells him this doesn't look good. Only time will tell. But Abbe doesn't like it, and she tells him so before breaking down again.

36

My body lies still, as though shattered by what it has seen. All about me is a jangled music of beeping woven into a liquid light, tainting all color that of the laboratory of Dr. Moreau. The scene isn't so futuristic as it is macabre. From out of my chest extend tubes that drain fluid from the hollowed pocket holding my heart as it quivers like a captive rabbit. Dave stands beside me looking profoundly out of place in street clothes, tugging on the long rubber tubes to produce suction, draw away fluid. He will remain bedside in the cool darkness for the next two days, personally guiding me through this trauma like a Cajun through his native swamp. This is Dave's terrain.

Abbe stands just beyond the doors to the ICU and calls on the phone for permission to enter. Other than having glimpsed my body as it was rushed on a gurney through the halls of the OR to the elevator, and briefly touching the chilled flesh of my forearm from between the hips of frantic doctors and nurses, she hasn't yet seen what they've done to me. The nurse briefly explains over the phone what she should expect to see, where she can and cannot touch me, and not to be upset by the battery of apparatus.

She approaches the doorway with short tentative steps as though her presence alone poses some unforeseeable risk. My body is horrific, my face, hands and arms blanched white, the skin swollen taut. The clear plastic of an endotracheal tube connected to a respirator plunges into the windpipe, while the body lies wholly supplicant to its steady wheezing, filling then emptying then refilling the lungs with air. The eyes are slit, the lids parted open from the swelling of translucent gelatin. They hold no light, no color, as they sit like stewed onions in the bone of my skull. The entire body holds a general yet acute expression of shock in its utter stillness, the complete absence of volition, desire or purpose in its dreamless morphine sleep. Soon there will be two realities: that which exists within and without the vault of my head. I should be dead and the body knows this. The brain, however, is snowed, and mindlessly prompts the organism to live.

Abbe's eyes are now dry as her head hovers above my face, about to apply a warm hand to my forehead, confident she won't cry. She has never much cared for crying, and has now told herself that this would have to be the last of her indulgence, at least for a while. Her fingertips cross my brow and she begins to speak with an even optimistic inflection, easy at first, then wavering, her voice finally drifting beyond control. Once her eyes fill it's all over, and she moves back slightly so as not to drip tears onto my tapestry of wounds. She collapses into a chair that sits just behind her, with her face in her hands. All the while she is oblivious to Dave's presence as he stands on the other side of the bed slowly, methodically, quietly drawing away fluid, checking my status minute by minute. He doesn't speak. His presence is inert but for the single-minded purpose of drawing life back into this half-corpse. When Abbe finally lifts her head and wipes the warm tears from her eyes, she sees his silhouette against the faint green light moving in silence, except for the rhythmic stretching and snapping of rubber tubes. She apologizes for crying and vows to pull herself together from now on. Her voice is hollow from crying.

He's doing great, Dave says matter-of-factly.

She stands and collects herself further, pausing before asking what happened downstairs. Dave relays to her the logic in the sequence of problems, followed by the sequence of solutions: the initial weakness of the heart, the bleeding, the swelling, then the slow steady improvement. He then conveys his typical optimism with his typical insouciance. Apart from insult to the brain, any damage done on the table is reversible, but of course nothing is guaranteed, he explains. All that he cares I do now is pee. So long as I continue to pee, he's happy.

He further quells her anxiety with his uncanny ability to make the extraordinary seem routine. He sees in her eyes that she is dangerously enthusiastic for knowledge of my condition, so he gives her some of what she wants. The drugs they administer to suppress the immune system are poisonous to the kidneys, he explains. So he'll be keeping a close eye on the toxicity of my blood as well. I will probably be in the ICU a few days longer than usual, but I should be on the transplant ward by the beginning of next week.

While they talk, my father and Joan appear at the foot of the bed. They too approach my side slowly, carefully bringing their quiet voices over my head, uttering encouragement to the prone and shattered body. My dad isn't quite so tentative, however, and comes right up to my side and whispers a prayer in Hebrew into my ear. Perhaps he more than anyone is heartened by what he sees because of his relative familiarity with such a scene. He mutters to Joan comparisons to Richard's case, and the fact that I look especially typical. What shocks others brings but a simple expression of recognition to my father's eyes. He and Joan stand side-by-side, making positive comments on the bizarre view before them, and eventually involve themselves in the conversation between Dave and Abbe. My father plies him with varied questions concerning when I'll awake, the chances of kidney failure, and what would happen in that case. Dave casually continues to work as he speaks. Again he is optimistic: he doubts my kidneys will fail altogether because I am still a young man. But if they do shut down, they'll simply put me on other immunosuppressants or dialysis until I recover. Also, he says, I won't be conscious for three or four days.

But as the week advances, the kidneys do fail. The combination of the marathon surgery together with the cyclosporine was simply too much, so a new plan is devised. The cyclosporine is to be replaced with antilymphocyte globulin (ALG), the very drug I had collected from the blood of horses twenty years ago. If I were conscious and if I were sane, I would see now the sunlight running laterally through the coat of the mare, see the broad horseflesh before me. Her serum now runs through me, keeping my body at bay. I must have known it would come to this.

During the first week of my stay in ICU there are no memories, only vague psychotic images. The family lounge down the hall, I will later learn, has begun to fill with friends and family from across the country. They visit me in an endless stream, disrupting the regular duties of the ICU nurses to witness my fantastically distorted body, my mad swollen eyes as they roam in their sockets, seemingly independent of the other. My uncle Irwin and Aunt Judy have once again come from Florida to be at my side, as they have for nearly every surgery.

From time to time I can make out faces I recognize, but the images become liquid, mixed up in dream and reality. I grow insane, I have no concept of time. All I know is that I am alive. I have had my heart cut out, another sewn in its place, and I am now alive. At least I strongly suspect all of this. But time and space begin to congeal somewhat as the effects of anesthesia and painkillers ebb. At a moment of particular clarity I feel a presence beside my bed and look over to see my father. He is holding my hand just as he had seventeen years ago. I have a sense of déjà vu, though I am cognizant of the reality behind the illusion, that this isn't a mere hallucinatory dream. He speaks, but his voice is muted by the medication, so I read his eyes. The expression is grave and confident. I want to talk with him, tell him I'm going to be all right. I am a child and my parent is here to care for me; it is my responsibility to let him know that I'll make it. So I try to speak, but can only produce a lurid moan with a trace of enunciation that merely communicates raw desire, an utterance from Frankenstein. I calm myself, lie back and allow the liquid images to solidify, the double visions to drift together, then I concentrate with manic effort. I grip my dad's hand and say through seized teeth, "The horse is BACK!"

The utterance elicits a whoop from my father. He cinches my hand in response, a signal I can comprehend. He has received his first message from beyond the grave. He bolts through the doors of the ICU to the family lounge immediately after leaving me and tells everyone what I said as he swipes away small tears. He and everyone else interpret the metaphor by empathetically placing themselves in my world of hallucinations: a large determined animal implacably lumbering around a racetrack, vision curbed by blinders, direction and will dictated by pure instinct. And they are somewhat correct. Perhaps I have managed to express instinctive will while my brain trips through this strange and terrifying world beyond the looking glass.

With the passing of each day my mind feels more stable, flight of thought a little less severe, consciousness more structured. I can now look over the crest of my chest and see the new scar that bifurcates the body, and how I have been prettily and properly stapled together. I admire the work when concentration allows. Sometimes I run my fingertips over my chest and arms, feel their puffed tautness in disbelief. What I cannot believe is that this body is mine, that these arms and this head belonged to me before the operation, my previous life. I slowly move a hand down into the groin and feel my immense, edematous scrotum that is now the size and shape of a catcher's mitt. This is not my body, I tell myself. This is another man's scrotum. And I believe what I say. Later in the day I will try to tell others what I think of this phenomenon, but they dismiss my lewd theories, not believing nor trying to understand me.

As the days flail by, their fatigued cadence fluttering unaccounted for by wandering consciousness, I descend into a private nightmare. As awareness grows, so does this harrowing sense of paranoia. The terror extends beyond the sensation of being trapped in a body I am certain is about to die slowly and miserably, and encompasses the knowledge that my mind is not my own, as it wanders aimlessly beyond the sympathetic boundaries that keep us all sane. The immaterial becomes material: agitation becomes a worm capriciously eating its way from ear to ear, a mad doctor, I am convinced, has transplanted my personality as if it were an organ. Sleep scutters by the doorway in a swirl of dead foliage, as the hallway has now become a brick street.

I haven't slept since waking from anesthesia. That was nine days ago, someone said, but I have no idea what nine days are. The temporal is infinitely mutable, I now understand. Days are nameless and always have been. But without a temporal framework I am lost, overcome with paranoia. Every time a nurse enters the room I accuse her of trying to kill me.

They think I joke. I tell one of them I can't sleep, and she mentions Dr. Llec, a mad physician and Vietnam veteran, a socialist, who specializes in sleep disorders. She emphasizes he is mad, utterly, totally thoroughly mad, and that this is clear to the sane. He is a medicine man dealing in nightshades, she says. Then her voice diminishes into a soft whisper. The moment she leaves the room he magically appears at the foot of my bed. Baggy fatigues cover his fantastically thin frame, a shock of white hair dances on-end over his brow like corn silk in a light breeze. I tell him my problem, how I can't sleep no matter what they give me, that they stole my mind and personality. He nods knowingly. I am trying very hard not to be crazy, I say. He doesn't reply, nor does he have to. He understands. Suddenly a cast of doctors and nurses gather at the door. They shoo him away with their arms extended, flicking their long bony fingers, taunting him with catcalls, cruel accusations that he is mad. I writhe about the bed, trying to speak, infuriated out of my mind. I am now convinced Llec's the only one who can help me. I intuit he is a genius relegated by the jumpy administration to crack cases no one else wants. Yet he continues to practice his very own radical brand of medicine with utmost probity and compassion as though he himself were a privy survivor of my very illness. Once he has left the room, the doctors form a semicircle about my bed and explain the method by which Dr. Llec induces sleep: he injects fifty cc's of morphine directly into the cerebrum. He is mad, MAD! they all shout in endless intervals. Out of this world MAD! Surely as a doctor you must know what this means? I understand, I say, demurely. And they leave, satisfied I no longer care to be placed in Dr. Llec's care.

I am now alone. The room is still, strangely quiet. In my relaxed dreamy consciousness I experience the pressure of a needle penetrating the skull, the cool compression of liquid filling the cranium, then the alternating sensations of heat and cold. I spin deeper and deeper into sleep, dreaming of sleep, immersed in its liquid warmth.

37

It is a private nightmare, a wilderness of mirrors. Friends and family intently conduct their happy lives insulated from the goings-on of a world disconnected from the neat fabric they recognize and nervously insist is reality. Only in brief flashes of terror does the subterranean reveal itself to Everyday Life, and only when accompanied by the simple universal catastrophes of flood and fire or dramatic manmade trauma. And of course the strain of heroic surgery can bring it about.

ICU psychosis, the phenomenon behind the debility, is common enough to have been given a name. With all the monitors reacting compulsively to every bodily function, the drugs that alter what is already a precarious emotional state, and the constant presence of nurses and doctors with the potential of bearing bad news, the psyche is overwhelmed. A grisly anxiety develops with the electronic beeping that corresponds with the pulse of another's heart, which you suspect upon awakening, is housed in your chest. The novelty itself is almost too much; the doctors have seemingly done this to mock nature or god with their precocious tricks. And what if the beeping stops? A ridiculous question to the sane. But to the rest of us the implausible is plausible, magic takes on the legitimacy of any law of nature. It is a parallel universe. An abomination appears, makes silent threats, then retreats into some shadowy mental apse, just as a doctor enters the room, listens to my heart and leaves.

A man by the name of Chris Eurich is somewhere here in the ICU. He has been here for a month, the nurses say as they speak among themselves. All day and night I listen to the musical wheezing of his respirator, the distant beeping of his equipment. From time to time I can hear the nurses asking him questions. The distance is an illusion, as he is just around the corner. When wakefully dreaming the noise floats into my room transformed as organ music, a somber Gothic tune of Ludwig van Beethoven. Eurich plays at a fevered pace, fluttering up and down the scale, his neck bowed over the broad keyboard of a pipe organ. Though I can't see his face, I sense perspiration collecting along his upper lip and brow, his mouth wrapped around the endotracheal tube, fueling the pipes with wind. He, like me, is mad, his music a mad expression of a mad composer. The tempo gradually picks up, batting like butterfly wings against the wind as the tune grows at once manic and precise. A virtuoso of immaculate precision.

Yet I can't take it. The music fills my mind, blotting out all other sound. I feel myself becoming lost in the melody, and cry out for it to stop. A nurse scurries in and I tell her to ask Chris to stop please.

"I'm losing my mind," I shout, straining for control. An awkward pause and I laugh gently.

"There's no organ in here, Bob."

"The hell there isn't. Just ask him to stop, please."

"I'll ask him."

But the music never stops.

On the wall at the foot of my bed I see large, almost lifesize pictures of Max and Miriam. They are vague memories of my life prior to this nightmare, Max sitting upright in the tub surrounded by soap suds; Miriam, with a large-brimmed reed summer hat. They seem to be guiding me through the wilderness, beckoning me on.

My stay in the ICU is extended a week due to surgical and kidney complications. All the while my ability to communicate with Abbe and my father are enhanced with time. Yet I am still insane. No doubt about it. I still can't sleep, the ceiling spins above me when I open my eyes to the darkness. Sleepless days become sleepless weeks. Dr. Llec returns in my hallucinations only to vanish before administering the morphine. And it becomes a Jewish wedding indeed. Faces are a steady blur, more like characters one might meet in a dream than creatures of flesh and bone. After two weeks of living among the real and imagined, Dave appears above my head, silently scanning the green figures on the monitors. He speaks optimistically of my numbers. I stare at the steady bobbing of his clean solid chin as he says I'm about ready to leave the ICU, ready now to head off to the transplant ward.

"Oh really," I say. My throat tightens as I keep my eyes on him.

"I think so . . . ." His voice trails off, his attention locked on to the monitors.

"Sure it's not too soon?" I ask, my voice laden with suspicion.

"Oh no. It's been two weeks."

"Well, I don't want to go if I'm not ready."

"You're ready." And he leaves.

I lie here, my eyes cutting back and forth across the hanging ceiling, my breath quickening. I'll die there, I need constant attention. One nurse, one patient. That's what I need, that's the deal. Dave's casual attitude is going to kill me. Perhaps he wants me dead. He knows Dr. Llec; everyone knows Llec. Professional jealousy? He knows this heart is no good, that I need another transplant. He's sending me to the operating room, not the transplant ward. He won't disclose this because I know his secret: Dave is really CIA. And he knows I am really Vietnamese. Beneath this fabric of skin lies a Viet Cong general, Ho Chi

Minh Pensack. This heart has turned on me, and now so has Dave.

The next day I tell Abbe of Dave's plans to give me another transplant. But she tells me that's absurd, that Dave had saved my life last week.

"Abbe, you just don't get it," I say.

"Bob, Dave loves you, I love you. The heart's doing great."

"He's brainwashed you. You can't see through his bamboozling.'

I consider her voice. She even talks now in Dave's easy and optimistic manner.

"Eventually you've got to assimilate yourself back into the world, Bob." She pets my forehead, curving her hand down my cheek as she says this.

"You've been talking with Dave, haven't you?"

"Of course."

"I knew it. He's got you snowed. You're all CIA."

Inexplicably this makes her laugh. In a privy tone I laugh right along with her.

The next day they load me onto a gurney and haul me down to the transplant ward. The sudden variation of new sights and sounds and smells is startling. The whisk of feet over the tile, the flood of voices, the odor of feces, the harsh light, a crying infant: the world has come alive. The composite of stimuli terrifies and exhilarates. All is out of control. Curious faces appear and vanish, the nurse's breath strikes my chest, paranoia rises up in me like a wave. I close my eyes in an attempt to collect my thoughts, only to be accosted by voices both real and imaginary. I convince myself to stay quiet, to hold on. If I maintain, if I stay cool and don't let the staff play with my head, the body will recover on its own, this edematous mass of water will come around.

The quiet contrast of the transplant ward is ethereal. As the gurney glides over the smooth tile I note the new Formica countertops, the fresh opal paint, the precise pastel trim rushing past, and I know that I am where they said I was going. My suspicion is eased. But nowhere are there any patients. (It won't be for some time that I'll learn these patients are too sick to be out and about, hence the ward is eerily vacant even to sane newcomers.) They unload me onto a bed, ask if I'm comfortable, and I lie, telling them yes, absolutely. Eventually they all leave but for one nurse, an Englishwoman about thirty years old. She very properly announces her name is Anne.

"So how many patients have you got, Anne?"

"Right now only two others." Her accent is heavy. She keeps her fingers laced before her as she speaks, as if preparing to curtsy when she finally leaves.

"If you aren't careful, you'll kill me, Anne. I'm really sick. Insane, too." I laugh nervously, then she does similarly.

"Not to worry, Bob," she says in slow, carefully enunciated British. "You'll be well cared-for. Now, can I get you anything?"

"Yeah. One thing."

"And what's that?"

"Can you make this bed stop spinning?"

She laughs rather formally, then leaves.

I march through the next few days sleeplessly, each endlessly blending into evening and night and morning; all the while the bed leads an acrobatic life of its own. Here on the transplant ward I have an overwhelming number of visitors, and I talk with them all, even if only to sidetrack my mind, to exhaust it. With each visit the paranoia is diminished, the bed slows.

I tell everyone I am out of my mind, that I'm psychotic, and they all say they understand. Bullshit. How could they understand? During each conversation I deconstruct their behavior, see very clearly how each personality is dictated by the owner's occupation. In my present mental state I'm sensitized, yet tolerant of everyone's play-acting. Each one of them begins to seem crazy.

As the days pass the personalities seem to grow more absurd, hysterically funny. Gradually it occurs to me that perhaps I've never been more sane. In spite of hallucinations, transgressions of the subterranean into the opaque realm of reality, in spite of the spinning bed, and cameo appearances by Dr. Llec, I sense a private insight into what's important, what I want my life to be about. I have retrieved a message from beyond the grave with my foray into heroic surgery, a message for Max and Miriam. It is a specific message, a code beyond the range of the written word. Therefore survival is primary. I realize this the day Abbe arrives with the children on the ward.

After a solidly conscious, albeit insane week of trying to understand and be understood by visitors, of decoding the language of the late-twentieth-century American professional, I hear the tapping of Max's and Miriam's small feet approaching down the hall. They appear in the doorway, hesitant at first, then bolt across the room and scramble onto the bed. Abbe tells Max to be careful of the tubes and wires, careful of Daddy, too.

Miriam can't quite make it up, but Max immediately curls his body into the small cove beneath my arm, his warm forehead against my ribs.

"You miss Daddy, Max?" I ask.

"Yeah." The word is drawn out for emphasis.

"Well, Daddy wishes he could play with the both of you." Never before have I considered play with such seriousness.

"We want you to be a horsie, Daddy."

"That's what Daddy wants to be too, Miriam. All Daddy wants to be is a horsie for Max and Miriam. Other than loving your mommy, Daddy doesn't want to be anything else."

At last, someone I can communicate with. Someone beyond the silliness of Everyday Life.

Then more contrast: the following day Abbe and my father are in the room while the bed is spinning like a carousel. I ask my dad to take hold of the bed, to steady it, and he does. I follow his hands as they descend into the mattress. Gradually the bed slows, and I thank him. The rational portion of my mind knows the bed is not really spinning, yet I see what I see, and it's a whirl of color. The bed is spinning. I am pleased beyond expression that he has done what I have asked, having believed what no one else has, and participated to a limited extent in this nightmare. But then he says emphatically, "Bob, *the bed's not spinning.*"

"The hell it isn't."

Abbe corroborates his story. "Bob, it's not. I'm looking at it right now, and it's not."

During the lunar debate, Dr. Moore, an old friend who is a trauma surgeon at Denver General Hospital, stops by to see how I'm getting on. The drama of the OR has gotten around. He's jocular, making concise witticisms about the doctor's life in an urban emergency room. But midway through the discourse I feel the terror of suddenly being trapped; social mores take on a new material dimension, become cagelike.

"I'm sorry, Gene, I can't talk now," I say, the feeling now drifting high up my chest near the throat. "I'm a little nutty at the moment."

"I understand, Bob." I'm sure he has seen this, being a surgeon of considerable experience, though he doesn't really understand. He has doubtless seen postoperative head cases many times over, but he could never understand. Right now I am insane in a way no one can comprehend, so I say with a baleful smile, "One of these days I'm going to terrify you all by coming to my senses," as if this were a threat. Unanimous laughter fills the room.

38

Perhaps it is the chrome frame jostling against the flanks of my bloated abdomen and thighs as Abbe propels me down the hallway. Perhaps it's the anticipation of direct sunlight. Either way I sense the resurrection of obscure memories, and the queer mixture of sad and ironic humor.

"I hope I don't cry."

"Oh, Bob, please don't," Abbe says as she negotiates through the crowded hallway.

An immense revival of déjà vu wells up from seventeen years ago. My first trip out of the hospital mysteriously produced tears, and I feel them rushing back now.

"I know everyone in this hospital. Everyone. I don't remember their names, but I know them and they know me," I say. My voice is fast and flutters like a schizophrenic's.

"You're still crazy, Bob."

"Sure am." I laugh maniacally. "But that doesn't mean I don't know everyone."

"Charming," she says through a smile.

More unrestrained laughter. But when the hydraulic sliding doors whisk apart and I am met with a cool breeze and the impact of sunlight against my face, the tears start. Within a short moment they become a hot brine pouring over my cheeks, accompanied by an unexpected rush of clear, simple thought and emotion, void of stray cognition or hallucinations. Amid the tears I lie back deep in the chair and allow the sun to strike my face at every angle, feel its warmth penetrate the saltwater rivulets and skin. Sunlight. Wind against skin. Sounds from the fluted larynx of tiny birds.

Eventually I try to stand, and manage a few steps before flopping back into the chair with the gravity and grace of a sea lion. After fifteen minutes the chill of the breeze sets in. Abbe maneuvers the wheelchair about, and we head back indoors. While waiting at the base of the elevator banks, Abbe mentions going up to six-west, the ward where I waited for this heart.

"You could show off your new physique."

"Reassure them I'm of sound mind."

"The nurses would be happy to see you. I think we should if you're feeling up to it."

Laura, the nurse I hardly knew and still hardly know, the receptacle of that initial gusto of emotion, stands with her back to us, her small hand madly scribbling across a clipboard. She turns, and, upon seeing me, shouts, "Oh, Bob . . . You're . . . here!"

"Yes, I'm *alive*." I say this with the mania of Dr. Frankenstein in my voice.

"And approaching maximum density."

I stand up long enough to take in her hug, then fall back again. Other nurses gather around us, ask questions, make ironic comments on my weight and wish luck. While sitting within the circle of voices, feeling tired and a little removed once again from the surroundings, a voice I don't recognize says, "Why you're *Dr. Pensack* . . . the man who received the last heart . . ."

I pivot the wheelchair to see a lady in her early forties with her hands to her cheeks gazing down at me in disbelief. The abrupt manner of the address does nothing for my paranoia that's now edging its way back into the day.

"Yeah, I'm Bob." I present her with a disconsolate smile.

"I'm Betty's daughter," she says. "We just received a call a few hours ago that they may have a heart for her." She pauses and shakes her head. "I can't believe you're here. . . . Would you mind saying a few words to her?"

"Not at all." I look up at Abbe. Her brow is widened in amazement. Betty's daughter also has a stunned expression, that of having glimpsed a paranormal coincidence. For me it is merely surreal and therefore quite ordinary. Nevertheless, donor hearts are true rarities anymore.

"She just received the call this morning?" Abbe whispers above my ear.

"That's what she said, right?"

"We sure did. The family is in the lounge."

Abbe hauls me along behind Betty's daughter to the lounge where we discover about thirty of her relatives anxiously watching a Broncos game.

"Everyone, this is Dr. Bob Pensack," Betty's daughter announces to the crowd. "He received a heart just three weeks ago."

I'm having difficulty believing this crowd is all of one family. The grip of paranoia makes it hard to breathe; cognition suddenly regresses to a Kafkaesque level. Again, that rain-splattered film has interspersed itself between me and the world. There's no communication, only random voices, random gestures, sound and fury. Once Betty's daughter introduces me, everyone stands, the television dies in a flash of blue light. Voices suddenly come from all directions as the crowd encloses, and they greet me as though I were a holy man.

"Hello, Bob, I'm Betty." The weak voice stands out from the others.

I turn toward it, trying to keep my head in the game. "Hi, Betty. I heard the wonderful news," I say, my voice hollow, foreign.

"Oh, you look like you're doing just great," she says. She appears grandmotherly, kindhearted, sensitive.

"And you're going to do great too." I stand up, walk over to where she sits in a wheelchair, and add, "I don't really need that wheelchair. I just wanted to go outside for a while, and now I'm a little tired."

A collective gasp is audible.

My mind is now focused on two objectives: not letting on to my insanity, or hinting at the shattering nature of recovery. What if I were to momentarily forget myself and blurt out that it's not worth it, that the pain and terror were too great, that they stole my mind, took my heart, that the procedure itself is barbaric; which is precisely how I feel in times of weakness—which is most of the time? Discretion doesn't come naturally at the moment. Is the reality of recovery a truth better kept secret? In spite of my present state of mind I feel an obligation to lie through my teeth, to provide this poor woman with the illusion of hope.

With a weary voice I give her sheer Pollyanna: "You're going to get your heart and do great too." When I hug her the hazel in her otherwise flat eyes lights up. Then, with my teeth set, I take a few torturous steps as an ostensible demonstration of my remarkable health as if it were nothing. Just before collapsing, I carefully, gracefully, and with supreme effort, sit back down.

The eyes of family members glisten, and Betty herself appears newly confident, downright certain of a brave new future. Abbe and I tell them all goodbye, and we roll out of the lounge and coast down the hallway to the elevator.

"I hope I did the right thing in there," I mutter to Abbe. "After all, I'm insane."

"Do you think cynicism is what she needs right now?" Abbe asks.

"It would be honest at least."

"Trust me. You did the right thing, Bob."

We head back upstairs to my room where I'm visited by an entourage of family and friends. But I'm not myself all afternoon—apart from my regular nuttiness. I'm especially quiet and removed from the discussion taking place around me. Everyone's nonplussed by my vacant mood, as my mind is on the ethics of the charade I just pulled. Also I haven't fully emerged from the clouded world of depersonalization.

The episode was bizarre not only in coincidence, but in its brevity too. It echoes forward through the evening with subliminal-like resonance. All day and night I feel I am trying to decipher whether it occurred in dream or reality. I am asked how I feel, what my plans for the future are, even when I will be returning to work, but my attention is hopelessly discursive.

That night it's confirmed I'll be discharged in the morning, though bloated and steadily leaking fluid from a lymphocele.* At home, Dave believes, I'll be able to sleep, the bed will slow if not stop. I'll grow sane. Though afraid for my life, of leaving myself open to deadly microbes and minor, yet fatal injury, I agree. Sleep and the promise of a clear head are supreme enticements.

*A lymphocele is a collection of lymph in a new surgical wound. They are especially common in wounds of the groin and armpits. After the transplant, the site where the balloon pump had been inserted into my femoral artery developed a lymphocele.

39

The wheelchair rolls smooth and quiet down the corridor. Above and behind me Abbe's and Dave's voices discuss a reintroduction into the world of the living with light humor. Through their conversation my mind feels as though a hummingbird is darting about the cranium. Their revved-up rhetoric is optimistic, quintessentially Dave and Abbe. Abbe remarks with incredulity that I've been within the walls of this hospital for five weeks now.

"That doesn't mean I'm ready," I say.

"Bob, you're only ten minutes away from us," Dave says.

"I don't know about this . . ." My voice has withered into a tired mutter.

The doors at the end of the corridor are a frame of incandescent sunlight. Traffic zips back and forth within the bright trapezoid of glass. My uneasiness mounts as the wheelchair inexorably approaches, driven it seems, by two people who simply have no idea how sick I am. Of course if there are two people who really do know, it's my transplant surgeon and wife. Nobody knows how insane I am, however. That's my paranoid secret.

When we get to the car, Abbe opens the door and I try to stand without Dave's help. In my corner vision I can see him watching me, his eyes on my shaking legs and arms, his mind in the process of reconsideration. When he finally does speak, he's hesitant.

"Now Bob, just call if this is too much too soon." He cups his hand into my armpit and hoists me up into the soft leather upholstery.

"Don't worry. I'll call."

"And remember, we want to see you here tomorrow morning at nine." The sudden concern in his eyes is unmistakable. I see he's serious and worried.

"You know, Dave, we have something for you. A little thank-you." I try to reach into the backseat but can't twist my blubbery abdomen, so Abbe searches for it. "You kind of remind me of a closet jock, Dave, so I thought a hooded sweatshirt would be an appropriate gift."

He takes it from Abbe and thanks us, visibly moved.

"Don't forget to keep your hands warm," Abbe says.

Dave pulls the sweatshirt over his head and stuffs his hands into the front handwarmer where he finds another present.

"A flask of liquor. Very appropriate for a transplant surgeon," Dave says.

"Don't forget to read the card."

He opens the envelope and reads the message as a smile works across his face. Then he pauses and reads aloud:

Dear Dr. Dave,
I was especially impressed with your ability to rise above your ethnic prejudice concerning my Vietnamese back-ground, and take such good care of me. I know there are those who believe my suspicions about you were delusional. But now that I am on my way toward recovery, I want you to know I still have my doubts. In any case, thank you for saving my life.

All my love,
General Ho Chi Minh Pensack

"I'm still a little crazy, Dave."

"I understand."

He carefully tucks the card back into the envelope, and asks if there is anything else he can do.

"You know, my skin is really killing me from all this bloating. I think the cyclosporine is making it especially tender."

"You need to fit yourself with a baggy new wardrobe. That's the only fix for now, Bob."

Just as I'm about to thank him again and say goodbye, I ask how Betty's transplant went last night. Dave hasn't mentioned it, so I assume it went well. After a strained pause, he says, "It didn't."

"What do you mean?"

"The heart was blemished, so we called it off."

"Uh-huh." I am unable to speak to this.

"It suffered some trauma in the accident, and it didn't appear safe to go ahead."

"You don't want to transplant a defective heart," I manage.

"You nearly learned all about that, Bob." He raises his hands in brief resignation to the reality of his profession. He then closes my door, and I roll down my window to thank him, and Abbe does likewise. The man doesn't have it easy, I'm thinking as we pull away. I watch his figure diminish against the immense white concrete of the hospital as the car is consumed in everyday city traffic. I feel myself slipping into a dark introspection occasionally encroached upon by the tossing of the car over uneven pavement.

"We should stop by the Cherry Creek Mall to get your new clothes," Abbe says after a spell of silence.

"That would be something to see," I say. "Me in a mall." My thoughts are scattered. I forget that this is my grand reintroduction.

But the experience really is something. Never before have I been in public in a wheelchair. It is a kind of admission of what I've been all my life—an invisible cripple. The mall is crowded with Christmas shoppers looking to buy a more natural-looking set of press-on nails, upgrade the china, investigate the awesome power of a La-Z-Boy. All the while Abbe is fantastically happy: I'm out of the hospital, she has her husband back, I'm not dead. Simple unimpeded glee. Yet I can't seem to shake this pervasive sadness, at least not until I feel seriously threatened by mindless holiday shoppers. My mind is with Betty as the crowd unwittingly threatens to overwhelm me. I imagine with terrifying clarity that I am a delicate soap bubble floating through a pine forest. A minor intrusion and my skin might rupture, the body fizzle into a puddle.

Abbe happily rolls me through the sunlit atrium beneath a canopy of indoor flora, past the glass elevator, the glitz of holiday window dressing, to a department store where we discover tent-like clothing that will adequately cover my sprawling flesh. She cloys me with attention, holding dozens of sweatshirts to my chest, careful of my wounds, her eyes taking in my new color. Her life has begun again, the crisis has been weathered. That's what her eyes tell me.

Once I possess an entire wardrobe, we head to the apartment where I will lie prone on the floor, my body swollen with water. Every few hours I take a light dose of diuretics that bleeds off but a fraction of a pound, or perhaps a pound, each day. And every day I feel I'm about to drop dead beneath the weight of this water. Meanwhile, Abbe floats about the apartment tending to the kids and me, gaily rushing out on errands, keeping the household operating. With the happiness that children innately bring to any home, and Abbe's doting cheer, a strange dichotomy develops in my mood. I sense the familiar presence of death amid celebration, like gas masks at a birthday party, whistling in the dark. The household has the paradoxical air of a Doors song, a fey melody burdened by melancholy lyrics. *Bloody-red summer, fantastic L.A. . . .*

My being home already seems brazenly reckless at heart, a kind of novel displacement, irony for the hell of it. While gazing up at the swirled plaster of the living room ceiling, I loosely imagine myself metaphorically: a pelican in Finland dying of frostbite, Trotsky in Mexico City, his chest holding an ice pick. Beware the communist who migrates south, and S-shaped bird that migrates north. At night the bed still spins, and sleep is as elusive as ever. The body feels corpselike with weight, while my mind is lodged just beyond the realm of the ordinary world.

As the days drift by the bloating doesn't diminish significantly, and I finally call Dave to ask what can be done. I'm drowning in my own fluid, I can't move, I tell him. This body is just too big. He agrees I need to be diuresed now that the heart is stronger. Shedding water is hard on weak hearts, so the process needs to be monitored carefully, he says. So huge diuretics are prescribed, the urinating commences, and the weight is shed at the rate of seven pounds each day. With weight loss I feel I'm now human again, more sure of survival. Simple mobility brings about confidence, and confidence brings about, of all things, sexual arousal of the most primitive sort.

Though I doubt it's ever been documented, I sense the brain damage I endured while on the heart-lung machine has radically lowered my threshold of arousal. My blood is summoned at the mere sight of my wife. I want her against me always, to feel her skin against my face and hands, her fragrance all about me. Smells have become heavier, touch more delicate, sounds richer. Every day I lie back on the bed as she hovers over me to cleanse my wounds. My hand is drawn to her cheekbones, down the curve of her neck, along the vertebral, onto her thigh. I note the tug of a button and the gentle strain of its buttonhole at the top of her blouse, and all I feel is sweet agony. She carefully irrigates my wounds without a word, carefully sets the dressings, then, once finished, places the material at the far edge of the bed. Then she reads my mind.

I look into her eyes, watch them roam along the scars, from wound to wound without any hint of revulsion or even shyness. She moves over me with care, gently taking me in, and I feel the weight descend. As the eyes dance across my shattered chest, I am thinking, Love spins a delicate yarn, a sturdy loom in pink and gold . . .

The dreaminess brought about by the narcotics erases the pain, while leaving the final sweet ache untainted. Afterward I am a new being. A part of me feels invincible and perfect, my mind awakened to a new clarity. I suspect I'll live forever. Of course my mood flourishes as it always has when confident of my health. I haven't made love with my wife for three and a half months, and I now feel a primal and visceral pride of having done so. I know the soft rapture of what it means to be a husband and father, even when the body lies fragile and broken. And so the days pass in a sequence of modest milestones, a sequence of private ceremonies.

Then one day I sit down at the dining room table after having fixed a small meal of minestrone soup and a salami sandwich, my body renewed with a wonderful appetite, a new desire for living. I watch the aroma spiral above the soup in a feather of steam, carefully observe the bread crust absorb the soup broth as I dunk the sandwich. My mind reels with anticipation. Then, with vague suddenness, I feel a hot wetness rushing out of the lymphocele incision and on down my thigh, as though I had spilled the soup in my lap. Relief, I think, a release of lymph. I stand, casually take up a napkin to mop up the mess, then pull down my new sweats, amazed at what I see: hot bright-red blood gushing from my ruptured femoral artery. I immediately know what's happening and stay calm. The first pulse you take upon entering a medical emergency should be your own, I rehearse to myself. I know I'm bleeding to death.

I shout into the kitchen to Abbe, "I'm bleeding in here."

She turns about to see the trajectory of blood squirting against the walls and ceiling as I try to plug the ruptured femoral artery with a forefinger. She shrieks, I tell her to stay calm, to try to find the phone and call Dave Campbell. After frantically rummaging through the house for the cordless receiver, she finds it on the kitchen counter and calls, only to reach his pager. Meanwhile my right boot is filling with warm blood, the walls are laced with rich crimson. After hanging up she calls 911 and summons an ambulance. Thirty seconds later the phone rings and it's Dave.

Abbe briefly describes the scene for him, and he asks if he can speak to me. Standing in a pool of blood, I take the phone in one hand while the other I keep tucked deep within the rupture.

"Bob, what's happening?"

"I've got a femoral artery aneurysm rupture where the balloon pump went in. It's a pumper here, Dave."

"Hang in there, Bob. I'll have the whole team waiting when you arrive at the ER."

Once I've hung up, I scamper into the kitchen so as not to jeopardize our deposit on the apartment. I'm also struck with the reality that it's five o'clock and the kids need to be picked up soon. Crazy thinking. I realize I'm getting a little shocky. This is it, I'm thinking. I get a heart only to die by a piddly-shit aneurysm. Already consciousness is fading. Yes, this is it, this has been my trip to the bitter end.

40

Time is dilated, accordionlike in its expanded progress. The paramedics have arrived without a gurney because, they will later explain, it was too long for the elevator. So they ask if I can walk, and I mumble yes, simply because I still can. While Abbe compulsively bolts about the apartment getting my things together and making phone calls, they walk me out the door to the elevator where I finally slump to the floor in a bloody heap. Consciousness fades, the bright cubicle begins to twirl in a whirl of light. Just as the doors ease together, I see Abbe's figure slip in between, then the floor lurches, gravity lightens. It takes Abbe a long moment for the ineptitude of the paramedics to register in the sudden quiet, as I'm sitting in a widening pool of blood, my chin nodding against my chest. One of the paramedics holds a white towel to the wound, and the terry cloth grows bold with red. He applies a general pressure, which isn't nearly as specific or effective as my own carefully placed finger in the rupture was, so the towel simply fills until it's saturated. What was something of a controlled bleed is now rampant. Once grasping the level of incompetency of these paramedics, Abbe goes ballistic.

"Why aren't you carrying him at least?"

They tell her to calm down, that the situation is under control. She's thinking, The Keystone Kops are going to kill my husband. This is elementary medicine. Then she begins shouting again until they whisk me away, and her voice fades behind the slammed doors of the ambulance.

All I see and hear are shifting bands of light and the shrill cry of a siren. In a brief flash of consciousness I gather we're moving, and I ask for Abbe. A voice tells me she's getting the kids. Unbelievable, but it has to be done. Another voice tells me they're going to try to get an IV into my arm as the ambulance bounces along. "Are you kidding?" I hear myself say. Then I pass out only to awaken a moment later to the snow of fluorescent lights as I'm finally floated down the hallway to the emergency room on the gurney that wouldn't fit in the elevator. I hear my condition described as being nearly exsanguinated, meaning I have nearly bled to death, then voices are brought up close to my temples. Jon Berman tells me everything is okay, they've got me. On the other side, Dave Campbell's voice tells me to hang in there. Suddenly a sharp pain leaps down my leg as the staples are yanked free, then, with a single deft and unforgiving motion, Dave tears open the incision that has now healed for more than three and a half weeks. Once open, Dave sticks his hand into the fresh wound and plugs the artery with his fingers. There's an incredible pressure coupled with the almost mystical sense that this is Dave holding on to whatever it is that binds body to soul with all his strength. I then hear myself shout, "You ripped my groin!" And I pass out.

I emerge from anesthesia with a shudder. The sleep itself is like a powerful dream I couldn't escape until there was some dramatic resolution to it. My eyelids flutter, batting away the residual fog of sleep. All light is dulled as though filtered through a weather-smudged windowpane. I realize I'm afraid, though I don't yet know of what. Then there's my father's voice through the ether, and with it comes memory.

"Bob, they did a great repair on your artery. You're going to be just fine."

A scene rushes to mind. An empty wall is suddenly braided with red lace, Abbe's face slowly shrinks away in horror, I feel my body weaken, a glowing energy cell dying deep within my chest. The scene causes the eyelids to tremble as I try to escape the mental scene. Then I'm struck with the pain in the groin; I can't feel my thigh and automatically assume I've lost the leg.

"I'm never going to recover from this," I whisper to my father.

"Yes you are, Bob. You have to."

I try to move, but quickly exhaust myself. Then comes the familiar tendency of the wounded animal to curl into itself. I'm crazier than ever, far beyond charted human experience. Just one goddamn thing after another.

Little changes during the long days of recovery in the hospital. Nights are haunted with nightmares, carnage scenes of the bleed, the surprise of sudden death. During the quiet night hours I want Abbe next to me in the same way a small child wants to sleep with his parents for fear of the dark. The surrounding emptiness takes on the form of personal threat, the threat of isolation, loneliness, death. Yet I think I'm now ready to die. For the third or fourth time in my life, I think I'm ready.

The daytime hours I spend learning about the three-hour surgery I underwent with detached interest, and what Abbe did and felt. As I suspected, the artery had ruptured at the balloon pump insertion site. Bill Krupski, a vascular surgeon, performed the artery repair, then took a thigh muscle and buried the ruptured vessel deep in the fold to provide a rich blood supply. That explains the grapefruit-sized bulge at the summit of my right leg. The wound was then left open to heal from the inside out because the method of controlling the bleed was far from sterile, with my dirty finger and Dave's finger sunk into the rupture for some time. Since my immune system is suppressed, the danger of infection is amplified. The wound curls away from itself like an enormous and gruesome pair of lips, a hideous reminder of what could happen again.

Once I was on my way in the ambulance, Abbe explains, she had to pick up the children at day care. Before leaving, she asked the apartment manager if he could have it cleaned before she brought the children home. Cost was no object; she just couldn't let them come home to this.

"Did you think you'd see me alive again?" I ask her now.

"I didn't know. Not with those stooges in charge."

I bring her face to my lips and kiss her forehead. Then I feel her face crying against my naked shoulder.

"You're a brave girl," I say, thinking: a familiar story, one I now see is taking its toll. Every time an emergency occurs, Abbe is left on the sidelines to cheer and pray, relegated to tying up loose ends. She keeps life civilized while her husband makes expeditions into the wilderness. A lifetime of near-misses. She cries now, her body quaking to pieces. When the tears dry and the convulsions diminish, we resume our conversation.

"So what did you tell Max and Miriam when you picked them up at day care?"

She wipes her eyes, her hands tightened into small fists like a little girl, and says, "That Daddy had a boo-boo." We both laugh at her garbled voice—my first laugh since awakening, she points out.

"When did you find out I hadn't bled to death?"

"At the emergency room. I saw Mike Grosso, and he told me he thought you'd be fine. But a few minutes later they paged me on the overhead, and I remember thinking, This is it. This is the moment in my life when they will tell me Bob has died."

"So where'd you go?"

"To the reception desk in the OR. I was afraid to give them my name, I was so full of dread. The receptionist's expression was so impersonal, so cold, I couldn't stand it. With hardly a word she handed me a bag full of your blood-soaked clothes and boots. A little later Jon Berman came in and told me you'd be fine. He doesn't candy-coat anything, you know."

I am quietly blown away. What a woman!

Two days later they wheel me out of the ICU, out of my familiar and terrifying recovery pod, to a general ward where I lie in bed in a constant state of anxiety waiting for the next event. Anxiety, however, is broken up by occasional mainlined doses of Dilaudid, a pharmaceutical equivalent of heroin. Once or twice each day I premedicate by pushing a dose-controlled button on an IV carriage, then go for a slow walk through the ward. My thoughts soar as the juice rushes down the mainline pike into my forearm. The horse is back, indeed.

When sober the pain is generally overwhelming, yet I gradually elect to deal with it clean, and sometimes even walk without dosing up. Then, toward the end of the third week it's agreed upon that I'm ready to go back home, as the wound is healing nicely, and I'm once again ambulatory, though barely so.

The ride of course brings with it haunted images, a quiet terror I try not to express. Winter has set into the city, trees are stripped bare, the sky is the color of gunmetal, yards bright with fresh snow. At home all evidence of the bleed has been scrupulously removed from the walls, ceiling and carpet. Being here, coming home, carries with it a traumatic memory, as though I have returned to the scene of a crime, a place where the integrity of my body and mind has been forever and irreversibly compromised. There is the constant reminder indelibly etched in memory of where I stood or lay as though within the lingering chalk lines sketched around a murdered corpse; the rooms are haunted by the ghost of my own body. I ask myself if I am dead.

And the nights are terrifying. There is no masking my fear and trembling. Where before I would pray, "God, if you're up there, go fuck thyself," I now pray for help. Terror has absorbed courage. During the daytime, Max and Miriam ease the anxiety with their uninhibited living comedy, their silly sweetness. My wife and children are the sum of my world; what goes on beyond the perimeter of these walls is of no interest to me. I am an island, my wife and children natives. I feel as though I am starting over now, ready to search, in meager ways, for the grace of god.

Four times each day my wife and I go through the routine of dressing the wound which involves removing the old gauze, irrigating the valley of the incision, then applying new dressing. The wound's gruesome aspect isn't something the children should see, so we distract them both with a game or treat, and disappear into the bedroom. Max is at the most vulnerable age, being old enough to understand what he sees as a terrible wound. If he were to see it, he might be terrified, traumatized by the visceral view of his father's anatomy. But one afternoon the doors silently pry open and Max's figure suddenly appears from behind Abbe, his eyes locked on the gaping wound, the pouches of fat and granulating flesh. Once I see that he sees, I explain that this is the boo-boo Mommy spoke of before. He isn't shocked, even very curious. Perhaps he has become accustomed to my chest that's laced with healed wounds, and happily believes that *all* wounds heal. At first he balks a little, then he says without so much as a trace of trepidation, "Cool cut, Daddy," before becoming once again distracted by the noise of the television.

4I

As the month advances, Denver grows oppressively ugly and its weather severe with hard winds that sweep over exhaust-blackened snow. A tiny white sun weakly penetrates the cold before collapsing in a small yellow flame into the mountains. Harsh, mundane and ugly. Meanwhile, Steamboat is receiving record snowfall, smothering evergreens from base to pinnacle in clean new powder. Privately I believe it would be good for Abbe, but reckless for me to be so far from the hospital so soon. Of course it's really not so reckless, as the doctors unanimously agree that a brief trip to the mountains would be therapeutic and nominally risky. But there is the burden of memory. What if I bled again and was hours from a hospital? Doubtful, so I decide to go, but more as a fuck-it-all gesture and disregard for this body, than simply for the fun of it.

So a few days before New Year's Eve we pack a few things together and are on our way as a family. The car climbs out of the gray urban snow into a pristine winter. Sunlight ricochets off naked mountaintops above precisely defined timberlines standing against a blue expanse. As we rise above the plains there is little of the anxiety I had predicted, only a strange exhilaration, a sharp thrill. Max asks bafflingly simple questions: "Why are there tunnels?" and I'm filled with the joy of communicating with a human being on my level.

As the highway parallels alongside the Blue River, the car

grows quiet, the children nod off to sleep, Abbe immerses herself in navigating the winding road. My mood grows contemplative, but not darkly so. A real departure. On the near side of a snow-field I watch a pair of Belgian horses trudging alongside a split-rail fence, the sun glancing through their honey-colored coats. Plumes of smoke pour from the doe-leather nostrils as they clod along vacantly, only concerned with maintaining warmth, locating food and water in an environment hostile to life. Their blunted senses seem to add a peculiar grace to their slow heavy gait. They are beautiful creatures with their short legs, thick bar-rel-like torsos and frumpy, womanly shape. They have no idea where they are, what pastoral scene they are the center of. The images return through the day unfaded.

Eventually we pass the Rabbit Ears and descend into the Yampa Valley where it lies insulated in white. The floor of the valley gleams in the late-afternoon sun, while to the north the smoked glass of distant gondola cars glints as they mount the spine of the mountain. This is all part of another world, I think to myself, one that couldn't be further removed from my world of hospitals. Impossible for one to imagine the other, and per-haps that's best. I try to imagine affluent tourists in Day-Glo ski suits riding to the summit where the comfort of the lodge moors complete with wet bar. There they polish off the day with decan-ters of Chivas and Stoli, and the pleasant ache of sore thighs as they lie reposed before wild yellow flames in a vast fireplace. The false sangfroid, the bravado, the ease at which laughter and for-getting come. Anyway, this is where I have arrived after three months.

The house couldn't appear more foreign when we enter and still be my home. I walk through the rooms as a visitor or thief. I recall the rooms, the design, the cherrywood cabinets, as though I had visited and revisited them in a dream. My legs ache from mild exertion, my breathing is heavy, and the hospital seems far

far away. However, I watch on, fascinated, as Abbe turns the children loose on the house, and they take to the stairway and sofa with such familiar purpose that I am reminded this is their home.

We unload the car, make phone calls to family and friends to tell them we're here, not so much with an attitude of triumph, but of daring. The next time I bleed to death, I tell my father over the phone, there won't be any deposit to worry over. Eventually we make plans for New Year's Eve dinner with friends at a posh French restaurant in Old Town Steamboat Springs.

When the holiday arrives I have my first shot of whiskey early on in the afternoon, feeling a sudden rush of confidence and health. Before coming here I had called the transplant coordinator, Karen, to ask if I could drink alcohol. She said, yes, but with extreme moderation. Is there such a thing?

That night I convince everyone at the table that there is nothing wrong with me, just as I've temporarily convinced myself. Though I'm easy on the alcohol, I attack the food with a fury, glutting myself on small portions of rich French cuisine. But when the dessert tray comes around, all arranged with elaborate cakes and pies, again I can't refuse. My voice and laughter continue to dominate the table until I feel myself tire, and I retreat into occasional quiet, staring at the slender candleflame within the glass chimney at the center of the table, my mind briefly capturing the moment and magically superimposing it against all I've recently been through. All day long I haven't felt the craziness, the paranoia, yet I've withheld the childlike viewpoint, seeing civilization as irrevocably absurd. That part of what I experienced in the ICU seems to have stuck. As my eyes follow the gentle wave of the flame, I wonder if I will eventually lose that too.

Without my voice I see that the atmosphere of the restaurant is rather subdued. As we get the check and prepare to leave I realize that I acted a little crazy tonight, that the contrast between my behavior and everyone else's has been noticed. Driving through the empty streets of downtown Steamboat, through what is a romantic re-creation of a bygone era and a culture that no longer exists, I ask myself if I'll ever assimilate back into the mainstream, and if I'll ever care to. This is the façade of the Wild West with a touch of Disneyland, a fabrication designed to attract the most circumspect tourists. This is a theme park, I remind myself. This is not reality.

Two days later we're heading back to Denver. The trip has been a success in spite of my condemnations; I am now considering whether or not I'm ready to return to stay. But just the thought makes me nervous, though physically I'm probably ready. The question of whether or not I can emotionally take being separated from the security of the hospital remains to be answered. After all, this week in Steamboat has felt like something of a spacewalk, a journey into more uncharted territory.

Tomorrow morning I have a heart biopsy scheduled, a bizarre and painful routine I now go through every two weeks. The procedure verifies whether or not the body is rejecting the heart, attacking it, and if not, then the doses of cyclosporine, prednisone and other antirejection drugs will not be increased. As time marches on, the intervals between rejection-free biopsies will be stretched to once a month, and finally every three months.

As a routine it is savage. A catheter is inserted into the jugular vein at the base of the neck, then threaded down into the heart where four samples of the startled muscle are bitten off with an alligator clip. Though the new heart is denervated (not a part of my nervous system), I can feel the sharp tug when the bites are made. This is part of the reality heart-transplant patients buy into in order to stay alive.

With each biopsy I feel the plastic tube floating down the jugular, then vanish as it enters the nerveless chambers of the new heart. I concentrate, try to control the very natural impulse to jump up and murder the most insensitive of the doctors. Finally I sense the tug of the alligator teeth snipping off tissue. After the four bites are removed, they will be sent to a hospital lab and analyzed under a microscope. If I am found to be rejecting, then the immune system will be suppressed with heavier doses of immunosuppressants.

But the following afternoon we receive the happy news of a negative biopsy. Yet already I'm preparing myself for the week after next when I go through the same routine again, with the wait, the dread, the anticipation of terrible news.

That night at the dinner table the subject of moving back to Steamboat comes up. We had planned to stay here another month, but when I mention the possibility of going home next week, Abbe's eyes brighten.

"This is the sixth negative biopsy," I say.

"What do you think the transplant team would say?" she asks.

"Don't know. I'll find out tomorrow." I stare ahead blankly, my mind calculating the weeks and days since the operation. "But I do know my heart was getting stronger while I was in the hospital after the bleed. It's been two months since the transplant. You have to take that into consideration."

The table grows quiet, our minds independently focused on the possibilities.

The following morning when I talk to Dave he agrees: in spite of complications, the heart has had time to become compliant and strong. But am I psychologically prepared to make the move? he asks. If I think my mind's ready, he's confident the heart is.

Of course this isn't a question I can answer yet. But by the end of the week I find myself surreptitiously bringing things together, modestly returning clothing to a parted suitcase instead of dresser drawers, imagining what it might be like without the emotional security of having the hospital just down the street. The playacting is a catharsis, all safe as make-believe. The week in Steamboat felt like an elaborate game of roulette, but the kids were happier and Abbe was beside herself. It all comes down to faith: do I trust this heart? The answer is: I don't know. Not yet.

But on Monday Abbe and I load up and drive two separate cars, each loaded until the wheelwells ride just clear of the tires. The drive is sunny, quiet and laden with apprehension. Going home. The ambivalence grows as the car progresses over each pass, out into the vast and snowy wide open of northwest Colorado. Springsteen comes to life over the sound system and suddenly I feel less fragile, more brave. The Boss. The cynical politics, the resonance of Vietnam, the lyrical myth of being tougher than the rest speaks to me. In the rectangle of mirror I see Abbe's car diminishing, then vanish altogether. The highway lies free and clear of traffic for as far as I can see ahead and behind me. I tell myself I am not scared nor lonesome, that the frozen landscape somehow isn't nearly so intimidating.

For the first few days we dig in and make the house our home. In the meantime I set up a cardiac rehab schedule at the local hospital, and within a few days I'm settled into a pleasant routine of mild exercise, rest and visiting friends. The days are infused with a pervasive exuberance, a pride of having survived. I am alive, I tell myself. Nearly every morning I awake with Max curled in the warmth between his mother and me, his small eyes lost in dreams behind the lids. I quietly slip out of bed into the chill and half-light and walk up the stairs with comparative ease to Miriam's room where she is stirring in her crib as she emerges from sleep. She is the daughter I haven't yet come to know; every morning we greet each other as for the first time. I firmly lift her up, holding her small lithe body to my chest, then bring her back downstairs where we lie awake together in bed, just she and I. It is a quiet and happy ceremony we languish in every morning before dawn.

While I've concentrated on recovering, Abbe has grown depressed. Now that she is home and all is quiet and settling into a natural routine, she has loosened her grip, let herself feel all those emotions that she wouldn't allow herself for the past three months. Now that the immediate danger is behind us, she has to dismantle her convoluted feelings that are a web of terrifying memories. When I come home from working out, riding the first of my endorphine highs in years, having reached a new plateau of fitness, she is sullen, always near tears. It is as though a brine of sadness lay just below the lower crest of her eyes, and if the surface tension is disturbed, tears spill over. It's a peculiar depression in that she's not hostile or mean-spirited in any way; she merely cries at the drop of a hat, she explains in the midst of breaking down over nothing. She seems frustrated with herself for crying and feeling with such incommensurate depth. I carefully try to explain it as a kind of reactive depression, a symptom of her own PTSD, a delayed response to all she's seen and been through. But I don't want to encroach upon her need to search out the root for herself. She knows what's going on, and doesn't need my professional jargon.

But her depression does hit me obliquely because for the first time as an adult, my body is growing stronger instead of weaker. I want to celebrate, to show a swagger in my step, the buoyancy of my heel. All around me I want friends while Abbe needs an empty house where she can let herself go without the restraints of etiquette. While our moods collide at first, I eventually ease up and give her the latitude and space she needs.

In the meantime I go out on the town with the giddy joy that accompanies newfound health. At rehab I work out excessively so that I might assimilate into a normal life sooner.

In the late morning I drive to the hospital where I work out on an array of peculiar machinery designed to test my new heart, make it strong and limber. I know everyone and they all know me. While working out I sometimes shadow-box with my shirt off, my fresh purple scars traversing the chest. A small crowd forms with their arms folded before them, repeating to each other what they all know: this man had a heart transplant three months ago. I smile as I duck and jab, wallowing in the attention and glory.

I grow a beard and let my hair go without a trim. A sea change is under way in my thinking, the earth has tilted. Everything is now seen from an original vantage. The hair and beard, I believe, parallel my new sensibilities of being a civilian, as opposed to the life of combat that used to be mine. The process has been fixed in my mind with the force of living allegory. The theater of war was the imaginary counterpart to my life, and now the war appears to be over. But it only appears so. Just as the smell of burning tires can hurl Vietnam war veterans back twenty-five years to where they relive the horrors of Tet, all I do is sense the silent pounding of this heart in my ears at night and I experience the trauma all over. Nevertheless the transplant has been survived, IHSS has been survived. It is now time to languish in the glory of victory. I am a civilian now. It is peacetime, détente.

With the assent of fitness I'm confident I will live forever. When merely maintaining a plateau, neither growing stronger or weaker, I slip into depression myself, filled with suspicion. I speculate about when this heart will betray me. So a few weeks after our return I go skiing against the better judgment of the transplant team. If I were to fall or get hit by another skier, my sternum, which is still sore and not entirely healed, could be seriously stressed or broken. Dave emphasizes that in such a case the danger can't be overstated. But I am cocky, and I need this heart to prove itself day in and day out, reassure me of its conviction and devotion. Every day I watch the gondola cars from the kitchen window, silently riding up the mountain; their flickering reflection of glass like small jewels strung on silver filament. Every day I wonder if it could be done. Physically, alpine skiing is an easy sport, as easy as you want to make it, really. But I am fragile. I own a heart of glass protected by a chest of papier-mâché, yet I'm willing to play the numbers.

Together Abbe and I choose a day and off we go in the car, encumbered with the precarious weight of ski equipment. Just walking from the car to the base of the gondola taxes my endurance more than I have dared try at rehab. The feet are frozen in boots that seize the ankles like a plaster cast, sending a flame of fatigue up my thighs. But anticipation keeps me struggling. It's been two years, back when I was in the process of dying. And I knew then that it could be the last time. Until now.

We get to the gondola with Abbe about to buckle beneath the weight of our skis, and me thoroughly exhausted. As we ride up within the quiet hum and suspended cushion of the gondola car, I look out through the smoked glass toward our house, the highway, the valley floor, and remind myself that I have survived.

42

Lights from headlamps of distant cars gleam in vague cones on the wet black concrete. The valley floor lies several hundred vertical feet below, spread out beneath the inky darkness. In the distance the low hum of a freight train engine mixes with the rumble of a thundercloud. The balmy air carries rain over the spring snow that stands in a moist blanket across the valley. For the past hour I've watched the subtle progression of weather, the pockets of silver and gold lights blinking in the distance while my family sleeps.

An hour earlier I was gradually awakened by a pulse in my ears. The acoustics grew louder, finally intruding upon a dream, and stirred me. I quickly recalled the dream. *I lie on the sandy bottom of a vast sea where the pulse of a passing sea horse reaches the shell of my ears through the saltwater. The muted roar, the red surge of blood becomes mixed up with rhythmic crashing waves against rocks.* Now, at four in the morning I'm gripped with insomnia, perfectly captive of the nocturnal landscape, fatigued by a long day of skiing. The impact of large raindrops against the windowpane eventually fills the room, smattering uneven at first, then developing into a torrent. Streetlights become distorted in the sheet of rain rolling down the glass, and the valley floor vanishes with the train.

I turn away from the window, quietly wander into the bathroom and flick on the light. I watch my eyes abruptly adjust in the mirror, witness the dilated pupils tighten into small black dots, then take off my shirt. For several minutes I stand before my reflection watching the faint pulse of this strange new heart in the mirror. There it is, suspended in my chest. The heart of another man. An alien heart. The pulse against my breast would be barely perceptible to any other eye, but I see it plain as day. I am acutely sensitized to it, yet I must admit I don't care to know much about its workings. My mood, my attitude toward it couldn't be more unlike my attitude toward the heart that now lies slumped at the bottom of two separate beakers, its unique anatomy being studied by medical researchers at the NIH and the University of Colorado Medical School. But that heart I knew. I felt comfortable tinkering with it. I could manipulate its behavior with the qualified assurance that it wouldn't stop dead in its tracks, though it nearly did on occasion. The fact remains that it *never did*. Somehow that heart was like a Volkswagen engine, something I knew well enough to tamper with and it would continue to run with mere gumshoe attention. It was reliable in its own way. But this new heart is of a different creature, a hybrid from another animal altogether, a cheetah or jaguar perhaps. It hasn't been mastered, and I don't know if I care to try. Yet there's this graceful throbbing I feel in my ears at night that I can't ignore. It lingers there as though my subconscious were constantly focused on it in the shadowy recesses of my mind, ever vigilant of the slightest stutter, waiting for it to abruptly stop.

The phenomenon is well documented, actually. Even patients who have had coronary artery bypass surgery have complained of pounding in their ears when they lie down at night in quiet darkness. It is an unconscious mental process at work. Suddenly the mind focuses on the rhythm of the wounded organ, and gradually the pulse comes to the fore. The sound fills the vault of consciousness until there is nothing else. Only the steady pounding of the heart of a cheetah. And here I stand watching the nearly imperceptible tap tap tap, and feeling the corresponding din in my ears. I take in my scarred bust as I stand naked to the waist. Here stands the body I was given.

Night passes. Just as the darkness over the mountains fades to violet, my mind quiets and I feel myself tire. I climb back into bed, feel the waist of my wife, and a moment later my mind glides again into dreams. A circus, a cabaret, intersecting jets of electric colors, and I arrive at the scene of an accident. The familiar cry of sirens is confused with the red and blue strobe; together they violently come at me. As I move toward the scene tears wash over my cheeks. I am told to stay away by an officer running yellow crime scene tape around the trees that surround a crumpled automobile. How strange. This is not a crime scene, clearly this was an accident, I explain to the officer. He suddenly appears suspicious. He walks up to me and eyes my face like a biologist studying a petri dish. Then come distracting sounds, concentric rings of light, and voices. Slowly, casually, I begin to emerge from sleep, bringing with me a fresh burden of contrition. I open my heavy eyes to find Miriam's face grinning, her forehead pressed against my brow. I see her new skin is smudged with wetness. No one has any idea where I've been.

The transition from morning to daytime passes in small episodes of family happiness punctuated with the cries of young children. The dream haunts the day like the presence of a friendly ghost. There is the air that something is about to happen or something unpleasant discovered.

Over lunch Abbe and I discuss plans for a vacation later this spring. We unwrap sandwiches from wax paper while our imaginations roam across the hemisphere—the tropics, the subtropics, Manhattan, then back to the horse latitudes. But in spite of the happy subject, the atmosphere is uncharacteristically somber. Abbe appears preoccupied and I occasionally drift off myself, my mind mulling over interpretations of the dream. Not that there are any dark and cavernous depths to plumb; now that this heart is finally realizing its promise, that it is becoming a part of *me*, I'm feeling guilt over the plight of the donor. Before I was either too sick to consider the delicate complexities of guilt, or growing certain I would die before a donor was found. I recall scanning the local news for accidents and suicides with emotional impunity for the most part. But I am better now. Midway through the Philadelphia cheese steak sandwiches I ask Abbe what's on her mind.

"I had a strange dream last night. That's all." She dismisses the subject further by widening her brows and listlessly shrugging her shoulders.

My interest is piqued. I straighten up in the chair.

"Me too," I say. "Mine had to do with a car accident."

"Mine was a trial setting with a judge, jury and bailiff. The judge had this enormous gavel." She can't finish her sandwich and begins to carefully wrap it back up in the paper.

"You really had a dream about a trial?"

"Yeah. We were both on trial for murder."

"The murder of the donor?"

"They thought we killed him for his heart."

"Seriously? You're not putting me on?"

"Of course I'm serious."

"It's just that it's such a coincidence."

There's a long refreshing pause.

"So your dream of a car accident involved the donor, too?" she says.

"I think so. I mysteriously arrived at the scene of a car crash just after the paramedics and police. They were taping off the area around the car like they would a crime scene."

"As though you caused the crash . . ."

"Exactly. As though I willed it." I study the Italian roll of the sandwich as though the key to the dream lay within the grease-saturated crust.

"But you weren't charged with anything?"

"No, but when I pointed out to one of the officers that this was an accident, he suddenly seemed suspicious."

"What did he say?"

"He didn't say anything. The dream simply ended. Suddenly Miriam's nose was against my cheek."

That afternoon we go skiing with friends whom I have little trouble keeping up with. Getting to the gondola is the greatest struggle, as usual, but once on the mountain I feel incredibly fit. I push myself a little harder with each fall line, stopping less frequently, letting the skis run and allowing my legs to absorb the mountain with an intensity that I haven't managed since I was twenty. There has been a clear breakthrough in strength and stamina during the last week. Perhaps this heart isn't bent on betrayal after all. Apparently it has taken to me nicely.

After a half-dozen runs I manage to get off by myself, peeling away from the back of our slow-moving pack after we make plans to meet at a restaurant deck in an hour. Cheeseburgers and baked beans in the sunshine are planned. But the socializing is getting to be too much. All day long I haven't been able to shake the residuals of the dream, nor Abbe's dream for that matter. I feel the need to be alone; my skiing lacks volition as my mind is elsewhere. I feel the skis floundering, so I cut through a grove of firs that blend into a grove of aspens, feeling the velvet cushion of new snow, then come to an easy halt in the middle of the forest. I look out over the valley and watch the traffic crawling along the shiny ribbon of compacted snow. My heart gradually slows as I stand in the sudden quiet. I watch the wreath of pale breath pour from my mouth, then, once I've recovered, I notice my hands are shaking. My eyes moisten unexpectedly. I feel something stirring inside, something like the need for meditation, prayer. Then I'm struck with epiphany. At the center of all this uneasiness is gratitude, not guilt. Guilt is easy, natural. A frenetic chuckle escapes in a burst, then tears gently break over my reddened cheeks. Astounding. After a moment of stillness the steady throbbing of the heart fills my ears, and once again I'm drawn back to the dream. It is the rhythm of the sea breaking against a rocky shore, corpuscles against taut eardrums, the emptiness of a vacuum. The understanding rises up in me like a hill. *Blood of my blood, flesh of my flesh, memory of my memory.*

After a long quiet moment the tears retreat, the noise in my head gradually empties. Sweat beneath my heavy clothing chills along the column of my spine. I slowly reach for the poles, stab them into the light airy snow, and once again I'm off.

On the deck I'm more reticent than friends and family are used to. It's a roving party with the sun gleaming through a tray of golden beer glasses as they are gracefully passed between shoulders. Every voice is loud, the laughter especially vigorous. This is what I may one day be a part of, I tell myself. Perhaps if I learn to repress the relentless intrusion of memory. I casually slide my hand down onto my groin where the femoral artery lies buried in a lump of blood and muscle, a constant reminder of the bleed. I feel its weight beneath my ski pants as I've found myself doing nearly every hour or so since the surgery.

The noise overstimulates me, bringing back the filmy window that separates me from the world. I want to isolate myself, think about the donor, my wound, our common fate. No one can comprehend what I've been through, nor would they care to, I'm sure. No one wants to consider the death of a donor in connection with my newfound health. Not on a sunny winter day. The average pedestrian rarely considers his own mortality until he is forced to toward the end of life. A certain degree of denial is necessary in order to live life decisively. Without it the idea of death consumes the mind, never allowing one's attention to focus on more blissful matters such as the lawn or manicuring one's nails, or even caring for one's family. Around me now I have friends who live more decisively than I could ever hope to.

The deck grows crowded with skiers in colorful and expensive gear. Fragrant white smoke rises off a long wrought-iron grate over a bed of glowing coals where the searing of ground beef fills the air. The atmosphere is decidedly festive after a winter of sunless days and constant snowfall. It is spring. I am a lucky man to see any of this. With that thought in mind, I turn to the crowd and propose a toast. Everyone enthusiastically hoists a clear glass of frothy beer above the table. The foamy heads pitch over the brim as I say, *"L'chaim,"* and the toast is solemnly repeated. *"L'chaim . . ."* I take a long pull until the effervescence fills my stomach, and my eyes glass over from the combination of emotion and carbonation. This is the life of laughter and forgetting. That's all I want. To forget for just a little while every now and then.

43

In the spring I gather my family and together we leave for Florida to visit Jimmy Tinnesz, the man I had spoken to over the phone the day I received the call. I feel drawn to this man, this audacious voice I have come to know. From the moment he opens the door upon our arrival at his home, there is an instant and magnetic bond. We recognize one another in the reflections of our eyes.

Jimmy and his wife, Gerry, have an eight-year-old son, Sam, who spends the afternoon playing with Max and Miriam. Though our families only spend the day together, Jimmy and I in particular find a friendship that I can only describe as incandescent in its intensity. We share our common experiences, our similarly altered world views. I tell Jimmy about my madness as a medical student and after the transplant, how I found everyone I met to be ludicrous, mesmerized with the pursuit of money and status, while they wasted their precious days in pursuit of both. He understands exactly.

Then two months after having returned home the phone rings at five in the morning. In my vague dreams I hear Abbe greet Gerry, then say, "Oh my god," and I am instantly alert. As I turn beneath the bedding I see Abbe's grave eyes, her unsmiling mouth. She blinks as though allowing a thought to register.

"Jimmy died last night," she whispers, cautiously handing me the phone.

In a shaken voice Gerry tells me the story of how Jimmy was feeling nauseated last night at the dinner table, how he suddenly went down on one knee before her and Sammy, how he then curled over on his back and his spirit slipped from his body beneath her fists as she performed CPR on her husband.

"I called because I knew Jimmy would want you to know," she says.

These words are flaming symbols in the eye of my imagination. *I knew Jimmy would want you to know.* For the next several months the news distorts my sense of orientation; I confuse my boundaries just as I confuse myself with Jimmy, Max and Miriam with Sammy. I meet with Bob House, a psychiatrist, and try to dismantle my sadness and fears. But it is something I know I will have to learn to live and die with, because there are no talking cures for such losses.

The following month another biopsy is endured. Again, no rejection. Mine is a textbook case, the surgery and bleed notwithstanding. Yet I recognize a pattern of anxiety developing through each cycle of biopsies: with the good news of each negative result, I believe I will be part of that 3 percent of transplant patients who never experience rejection. Then after a week worry settles in, imperceptibly at first, like a cat. As the date of the next biopsy approaches I convince myself that my body began attacking the heart with a fever just as I left the hospital the last time. The reality is that you can feel fine while experiencing life-threatening rejection. You need a hospital to tell you what is going on with your heart. There is still the anxiety of being far from the secure society of doctors and nurses. As the biopsies grow less frequent with time, the discipline required to remain poised and confident becomes exponentially greater. I am coming to realize that to perform simple tasks without the preoccu-

pation of this invisible illness haunting every motion is gone forever.

This last time the biopsy took three times as long as usual due
to difficulty in biting off four usable samples. My father came
down to Denver with me and watched on, all the while not saying a word, his body rigid with every gasp of pain and fear I
released as an echo into the laboratory. Once the procedure was
finally complete, he was unusually reserved. Here was a dramatic
reminder of the new set of harsh realities I now live with. I am
not all better now as everyone, myself included, would like to
believe. My life now depends on the doctors' ability to solve a
complex series of problems. But I continually remind myself
that the body is a problem for all human beings, that in this
respect I am not unique. Life is what occurs when the body is
well.

We have a full agenda for our weekend together in Denver. I
brought Dad down with me for a thorough checkup. For the past
two weeks there have been subtle signs of apprehension from
him concerning his health. At seventy-two, he worries about
cancer. The subject has surfaced unexpectedly, followed by a
quiet dwelling. We talk about it for a while, and the subject
vanishes as unexpectedly as it appeared. Gradually he is being
introduced into the terrifying world I've come to know so intimately. My heart goes out to him. So I set him up with the best
and have him rigorously tested only to discover everything is
fine. In the face of good news, I feel a certain pride, a son's pride,
of tending to my father's needs with respect to my profession. I
want to show him the neighborhood, small ways to cope, battle
tactics. Throughout the weekend his company has moved me
unexpectedly; we talk with more immediacy and compassion for
each other than we ever have.

I have an appointment with Bob House in a half hour, I tell

him as we drive away from the hospital after the biopsy. I ask if he'd like to sit in. I tell him Bob asked last week if I would mind answering the questions of a few University of Colorado medical students concerning my recovery and life as a patient and doctor. I make it clear that he wouldn't be the only one. "You bet," he says, genuinely curious about what goes on during these mysterious sessions. Perhaps to him they were once an exchange of arcane ideas and emotions, ungrounded in any meaningful way to what goes on in the ordinary world. But not now, not today.

As we drive I look over at his slightly shrunken figure, the crow's-feet imbedded into the temples, the profile of his eyes when he is sanguine and content. My mind suddenly rushes backward. *They tell me they have a new heart for me and it's only twenty years old, the body is a problem that can now be solved.*

We pull into the parking lot before the short brick of the psychiatry building where I started my residency nearly eight years ago. We walk beneath the flat overcast skies, through the humid and fragrant spring air, into Bob's office where a semicircle of students politely sits on the sofa.

Since Dad and Bob met one another at the time of my transplant, the introduction is brief. The exchanges continue around the half-circle of students, the atmosphere is subdued through the preliminaries, and not until we seat ourselves and Bob asks me to tell them a bit about myself does the burden of propriety lift. I immediately put them at ease with an explosion of jokes.

A random narrative develops, and I begin to mix in factual details that have little or nothing to do with why we're all here together. The jokes become rapid-fire, the familiar pose of nonchalance that I so easily assume when nervous or concealing private pain. As the questions come at me, I at once parry them with witty remarks until the initial inquiry is unrecognizable.

Then my father breaks in.

"Excuse me, Bob," he begins, addressing Bob House, not me. His voice carries the authority of someone who has something to say and isn't going to leave until it has been said.

"I don't think anyone can comprehend what Bob's been through. And I think it's hard for him to try and share fragments and pieces of it with people he doesn't know well. A little more than an hour ago he was lying on a surgical table in a heart cath lab a few blocks away and having four bits of his heart snipped off. After an hour and a half of that, he pulled his shirt back on and came here." He pauses. I see the muscles in his neck redden with this unusual display of conviction. It is also unusual—no, unprecedented—that my father has felt the need to speak for me. I sit back in startled silence.

"Bob's lived with this disease since he was fifteen. Since then, through all the surgeries, through the transplant and the recovery, they've broken him—his spirit, his body, his mind—and left it up to him to put it all back together. And I think that's what you're witnessing now. You're seeing Bob trying to keep it all together through humor."

I watch his profile as he makes this speech. Small tears have swollen and spilled over the wrinkled lower lids, his posture has become erect with urgency. These are the first tears of his I've seen since I was a boy.

Once he has finished, a pall of silence descends over the room. I keep my eyes on my dad until Bob House's voice breaks the quiet, then feel my hand float over to his thigh and tighten about the tense muscles.

The remaining time is a frantic exchange of revealing questions and answers. The meeting is salvaged from the wreckage. The students are clearly struck by the sudden frankness of my answers.

The following afternoon at the hotel room we receive the news that was both hoped for and expected. No rejection, I'm free to leave town anytime. During the drive home my father and I talk about the session, how he felt he needed to speak up. The conversation unwinds into how this disease has affected his life. He has lived with death haunting his family for thirty-eight years now, and never once has he been able to simply put it aside, allow himself the luxury of living beyond its domain. He innocently married a woman, whom he had two children by, then this. The mysterious union of blood and memory has bound him to it regardless, and meanwhile, there has been a life demanding to be lived.

"It's been a tough row to hoe, Dad," I tell him during a pause in our conversation.

"Yeah. Yeah it has. But apart from your mother, we've survived."

"I meant for you. You've had it tough."

"Well . . ." and his voice sputters. In many ways he is a modest man, someone who simply does not accept self-pity.

We arrive in Steamboat near dusk. At the end of the valley the sun has sunk below the hills and is throwing up a brilliant spectrum of amber that fades into the deep blue night sky. The household is quiet when I appear through the front door, but gradually becomes excited for a time before quieting again. I set my dop kit down, close the door, then allow my muscles to recover from the stairs.

"So you won't have to leave again, Daddy?" Max asks.

"No, I've got to keep going down there, but not as often, Max."

"To see Dr. Dave?"

"Dr. Dave and Dr. Bob. Those are the two guys who keep me together."

A lost look fills his eyes.

"Who's Dr. Bob?"

"A psychiatrist, like your daddy."

Another lost expression.

I kiss Abbe and hand her a potted plant with a note wedged within the slender stems I bought in Denver. She tells me the kids have been fed and are tired from a hard day at play. Miriam has nodded off to sleep under the coffee table with her bottle cocked into the corner of her mouth like a drunken hobo. In her arm she clutches her polar bear; she is now equipped for a long journey through a fantastic world of infant dreams.

That evening Abbe and I stay up late into the night. I tell her about the biopsy, the meeting with Bob, our drive home. She is quietly amazed. The conversation is light and peaceful in a way that was never possible before. She tells me about her weekend, about messages left by the hospital who is still owed by the insurance company, and a brief plea from a drug company who supplies the cyclosporine and also hasn't yet seen a dime. Intrusions of the outside world. Right now they do not exist. Right now I am listening to my wife who, like me, is ultimately unconcerned with the mechanics of what goes on beyond the walls of our home. She clearly doesn't broach the subject to spoil the quiet mood. Upstairs Max and Miriam sleep, by morning they will be as close as lovers. This is my family, I tell myself, this is my domain. I remind myself of the importance of survival and of simple living. Because with my family I am saved.

Abbe yawns and pulls her thick dark hair from her eyes. I reach over and pull her into my arms and hold her there, kissing her forehead. Eventually we wander off to bed, and for the first time in a long time, sleep comes easily. I struggle to ward it off for a few moments because I'm not certain I want the day to end just yet. This is not mere insomnia, fear of closing my eyes and careening into dreams, or fear of never waking up. It has simply been a good day. After a few moments I carefully crawl out of bed and wander toward the bathroom to watch my heart again in the mirror. The evening air is warm and balmy, the house quiet and lit with refracted moonlight. As I step into the living room I hear little feet coming down the staircase, then Max's voice whispers my name. From between the log banister rails I see his tiny figure in the gray light.

"Daddy," he says again, his voice now a loud whisper.

"Yeah, Max?"

"I want to ask you a question."

"What is it, Maxie?"

He lumbers down the staircase, the individual steps that are nearly too much for his small legs. As he approaches me, I squat so that we're looking each other in the eye. He takes a deep breath and speaks:

"Are you all better now?"

"Yeah, Maxie. I am."

"Can I listen to your new heart?"

"Sure." I saunter into the bedroom and pull out a stethoscope curled in a reed basket on the dresser, then quietly walk out without waking Abbe. In the living room I lie down on the sofa and Max climbs onto my chest. He curls his body into the shape of a shell and I gently pull apart the chrome tubes that gracefully bow into earpieces, and lower them over his delicate head.

"Does that feel all right, Max?" I ask.

He nods.

I take the sensor of the stethoscope and hold its cool metal mass to my naked chest and ask if he hears anything. He waves his head, so I slowly float the disk across my chest. Finally he nods yes. He hears it. My new heart echoes in his small ears, his nascent memory. I inhale deeply a few times and he nods again like a true professional, then pries the stethoscope from his ears and says, "Sounds really good, Daddy."

"Good, Maxie. I'm glad it sounds good to you."

I set the stethoscope on the coffee table and wrap my arms about his small compact body. Within a minute or two I am holding the steady rhythmic breathing of his sleeping body to my chest. I shift about on the cushions and see his mouth stretch open and release a yawn. Outside I sense it's about to rain. A sudden buckle in the wind heaves against the house. Here I am. The wind presses against the windowpane smearing it with a fine rain. The moon vanishes behind dense low clouds. I feel the approach of sleep and allow my mind to stray into dreams. I imagine now that if I were to walk out into the silver gray light, into that imaginary space where all things are equally possible and impossible, practicable and impracticable, all I would see before me is road.

AFTERWORD

Since his transplant, Bob has had recurring episodes of rejection, which were treated with increased doses of prednisone. Shortly after this treatment began, Bob became euphorically manic and painted the interior of his garage red. Subsequent increases in prednisone, however, have been less pleasant, as they have brought on episodes of mental confusion, anxiety, and diabetes. After his fifth positive biopsy, he went to Pittsburgh and met his old friend Dr. Starzl, and with his help he was placed on an alternative immunosuppressant called FK-506. For the time being, Bob's biopsies have been rejection-free, his diabetes continues to fade, and he has regained much of the strength lost through the series of rejections.

Richard's has been a success story, as his biopsies continue to be rejection-free three years after his transplant. But his oldest son, Benjamin, no longer plays basketball due to the symptoms of IHSS, and his younger fourteen-year-old son, Adam, still hasn't been diagnosed. This is the meager consolation of the family. Richard still views himself as a lucky man: he has his sons and he has his faith.

What lies ahead for Bob's children, presently age five and three respectively, remains to be seen. He plans to spend the lion's share of his time with his wife Abbe, Max and Miriam in Steamboat Springs, Colorado.

ABOUT THE AUTHORS

Robert Jon Pensack, M.D., is a general practitioner and psychiatrist. He was raised in Livingston, New Jersey. He received his Bachelor of Arts and Medical Degree from the University of Colorado, where he also completed his training. He now serves on the board of directors of the Transplant Recipients International Organization (TRIO) and lives with his wife, Abbe, and two children, Max and Miriam, in Steamboat Springs, Colorado.

Dwight Arnan Williams was raised in Princeton, Illinois, and now lives in Steamboat Springs, Colorado. He attended the University of Iowa and the University of Colorado at Boulder, where he was the recipient of a Jovanovich Award for his short fiction.

TO REMEMBER ME

The day will come when my body will lie upon a white sheet neatly tucked under four corners of a mattress located in a hospital busily occupied with the living and the dying. At a certain moment a doctor will determine that my brain has ceased to function and that, for all intents and purposes, my life has stopped.

When that happens, do not attempt to instill artificial life into my body by the use of a machine. And don't call this my deathbed. Let it be called the Bed of Life, and let my body be taken from it to help others lead fuller lives.

Give my sight to the man who has never seen a sunrise,
a baby's face or love in the eyes of a woman.

Give my heart to a person whose own heart has caused
nothing but endless days of pain.

Give my blood to the teen-ager who was pulled from the wreckage
of his car, so that he might live to see his grandchildren play.

Give my kidneys to one who depends on a machine to
exist from week to week.

Take my bones, every muscle, every fiber and nerve in my body
and find a way to make a crippled child walk.

Explore every corner of my brain. Take my cells, if necessary,
and let them grow so that, someday, a speechless boy will shout at
the crack of a bat and a deaf girl will hear the sound of rain
against her window.

Burn what is left of me and scatter the ashes to the winds
to help the flowers grow.

If you must bury something, let it be my faults, my weaknesses
and all prejudices against my fellow man.

Give my sins to the devil.

Give my soul to God.

If, by chance, you wish to remember me, do it with a kind
deed or word to someone who needs you.
If you do all I have asked, I will live forever.

—WRITTEN BY ROBERT N. TEST

"To Remember Me" reprinted courtesy of The Living Bank, P.O. Box 6725, Houston, TX 77265. (1-800-528-2971) Previously printed in the *Cincinnati Post*; reprinted in *Reader's Digest*; appeared in Dear Abby's syndicated column December 1977.